TOLERANCES
An Orthopaedic Reference Manual

second edition

TOLERANCES
An Orthopaedic Reference Manual

second edition

Scott Nelson, MD
Assistant Clinical Professor
Department of Orthopaedic Surgery
Loma Linda University

Montri Wongworawat, MD
Assistant Professor
Department of Orthopaedic Surgery
Loma Linda University

Loma Linda University Press

Nelson, Scott, 1970-
  Tolerances : an orthopaedic reference manual / authors, Scott Nelson, Montri Wongworawat.-- 2nd ed.
     p. ; cm.
  Includes bibliographical references.
  ISBN 1-59410-009-8 (alk. paper)
  1. Orthopedics--Handbooks, manuals, etc. 2. Musculoskelatel system--Physiology--Handbooks, manuals, etc. 3. Musculoskeletal system--Wounds and injuries--Handbooks, manuals, etc.   I. Wongworawat, Montri, 1973- II. Title.
  [DNLM: 1. Orthopedic Procedures--methods--Handbooks. 2. Musculoskeletal Physiology--Handbooks. 3. Musculoskeletal System--injuries--Handbooks. 4. Physical Examination--standards--Handbooks. 5. Wounds and Injuries--classification--Handbooks. WE 39 N431 2005]
  RD732.5N45 2005
  616.7--dc22
                                        2005028853

**"Never memorize anything
you can look up."**

- Albert Einstein

WARNING

The information contained in this book can be very dangerous if used inappropriately and is intended for use by those with experience in orthopaedics. The tolerances, indications and classifications presented in this book have been extracted from a number of well respected textbooks and journals with which the user of this guide should be familiar. The author gives no recommendations as to *when* an indication or tolerance is appropriate. Certainly these numbers are not appropriate for every situation. Patient factors, geographic location, timing, stage of healing, associated injuries, surgeons skill, and equipment available are some of the many factors that must be considered by the practitioner when using this guide to make treatment decisions. The maximum acceptable tolerances listed herein are not meant to define how much laziness a surgeon can get away with. They are meant to be used as a guide to help competent orthopaedic surgeons make clinical decisions which will most benefit the patient. The author cannot accept any responsibility for the inappropriate use of the tolerances and indications cited.

This book was created for boneheads who occasionally forget numerical tolerances of fracture acceptability, complex classification schemes, and other important and unimportant orthopaedic trivia. For those who like to quote "the literature" this book will enable them to do it with precision. And for those who have to listen to people quoting "the literature" this book will enable them to abort the propagation of erroneous numerical data.

TABLE OF CONTENTS

PREFACE

Christopher Jobe, M.D.
Professor and Chairman
Department of Orthopaedic Surgery
Loma Linda University School of Medicine

Five years ago, Scott Nelson, M.D., and Montri Wongworawat, M.D., brought out their first edition of this small, but information packed, text. As time has moved on and orthopaedic knowledge has been developed, changes have occurred, as might be expected, in the exact numbers of the tolerances and indications. These changes call for a new edition. In that same period of time, experience with use of this text has been gathered, and the text is more useful than ever. In this preface I would like to re-emphasize the importance of this text for the more experienced orthopaedic resident and surgeon. The experienced surgeon understands not only the principles of treatment but has been around for some of the evolutions of the tolerances. This small text places at his or her fingertips the most recent tolerances and indications so that they may be applied in short order in treatment. This has certainly been true in my own practice. I still have my original copy of Tolerances & Indications that I have found extremely useful over the past five years.

May 31, 2005

EDITORIAL STAFF

Antony Boody, M.D.
Resident, Department of Orthopaedic Surgery, Loma Linda University Medical Center

James Boyd, M.D.
Resident, Department of Orthopaedic Surgery, Loma Linda University Medical Center

Sean Hassinger, M.D.
Resident, Department of Orthopaedic Surgery, Loma Linda University Medical Center

Jonathan King, M.D.
Orthopaedic Associates of Coeur d' Alene, Idaho

John Schlechter, D.O.
Resident, Department of Orthopaedic Surgery, Riverside County Regional Medical Center

REFERENCES

BD   Bridwell KH and Dewald, eds. *Textbook of Spinal Surgery*. 2nd ed. Philadelphia, PA: Lippincott Williams & Wilkins; 1997.

BJ   Browner BD, Jupiter JB, Levine AM, Trafton PG. *Skeletal Trauma: Basic Science, Management, and Reconstruction*. 3rd ed. Philadelphia, PA: Saunders; 2003.

C   Canale ST, ed. *Campbell's Operative Orthopaedics*. 10th ed. Philadelphia, PA: Mosby; 2003.

CH   Chapman MW, ed. *Chapman's Orthopaedic Surgery*. 3rd ed. Philadelphia, PA: Lippincott Williams & Wilkins; 2001.

G   Green DP, Hotchkiss RN, Pederson WC, and Wolfe SW, eds. *Green's Operative Hand Surgery*. 5th ed. Philadelphia, PA: Churchill Livingstone; 2005.

GS   Green NE and Swiontkowski MF. *Skeletal Trauma in Children*. 3rd ed. Philadelphia, PA: Saunders; 2003.

HSU   Trumble TE, ed. *Hand Surgery Update 3*. Rosemont, IL: American Society for Surgery of the Hand; 2003.

LW   Morrissy BT, ed. *Lovell and Winters' Pediatric Orthopaedics*. 5th ed. Philadelphia, PA: Lippincott Williams & Wilkins; 2000.

OKU7   Koval KJ, ed. *Orthopaedic Knowledge Update 7*. Rosemont, IL: American Academy of Orthopaedic Surgeons; 2002.

OKU8   Vaccaro AR, ed. *Orthopaedic Knowledge Update 8*. Rosemont, IL: American Academy of Orthopaedic Surgeons; 2005.

OKUFA   Richardson EG, ed. *Orthopaedic Knowledge Update: Foot and Ankle 3*. Rosemont, IL: American Academy of Orthopaedic Surgeons; 2003.

OKUHKR   Garvin K, Pellicci PM, and Tria AJ, eds. *Orthopaedic Knowledge Update: Hip and Knee Reconstruction 2*. Rosemont, IL: American Academy of Orthopaedic Surgeons; 2000.

OKUP   Sponseller PD, ed. *Orthopaedic Knowledge Update: Pediatrics 2*. Rosemont, IL: American Academy of Orthopaedic Surgeons; 2002.

OKUT   Kellam JF, Fischer TJ, Tornetta P, et al. *Orthopaedic Knowledge Update: Trauma 2*. Rosemont, IL: American Academy of Orthopaedic Surgeons; 2000.

OKUSpt   Arendt EA, ed. *Orthopaedic Knowledge Update: Sports Medicine 2*. Rosemont, IL: American Academy of Orthopaedic Surgeons; 1999.

OKUSpine Fardon D, Garfin S, ed. *Orthopaedic Knowledge Update: Spine 2*. Rosemont, IL: American Academy of Orthopaedic Surgeons; 2001.

RG   Bucholz RW and Heckman JD, eds. *Rockwood and Green's Fractures in Adults*. 5th ed. Philadelphia, PA: Lippincott Williams & Wilkins; 2001.

RWB   Beaty JH and Kasser JR, eds. *Rockwood and Wilkins' Fractures in Children*. 5th ed. Philadelphia, PA: Lippincott Williams & Wilkins; 2001.

ADULT TOLERANCES

Transfusion indications and risks *OKU8-176, OKUHK57*
>One unit PRBC should increase hgb by 1.0 g/dl (hct 3%)
>Indications
>>Hgb < 6 g/dl
>>Hgb 6-10 g/dl with significant history of cardiovascular disease
>>Erythropoietin indicated for patients with preoperative hgb 10-13 g/dl ▶ 600 U/kg SQ on preoperative days 21, 14, 7, and day of surgery
>Risks
>>HIV = 1/200,000 to 1/2,000,000
>>Hep C = 1/30,000 to 1/150,000
>>Hep B = 1/30,000 to 1/250, 000
>>HTLV = 1/641,000
>>Bacteria = 1/500,000
>>Death from driving a car = 1/1,000,000

Radiation Risk *LW91*
>Background radiation in the US = 300 mrem/year (cosmic radiation, radioactive deposits on earth's surface, radon gas, etc.)
>Adult CXR = 15-20 mrem
>AP pelvis = 100 mrem (equivalent to 4 months of background radiation)
>CT abdomen and pelvis = 1,350 mrem (equivalent to 4.5 years of background radiation)

General

Open fx classification *JBJS 1976;58A:453*
  Grade I
    < 1 cm long wound
    low energy
    bone piercing from inside out
    minimal soft tissue injury
  Grade II
    wound 1-10 cm long
    moderate soft tissue injury
  Grade IIIa
    high energy
    wound usually > 10 cm
    extensive soft tissue devitalization
  Grade IIIb – inadequate soft tissue coverage
  Grade IIIc – associated vascular injury
  Special situations (upgrades to a Grade III)
    Shotgun wound
    High-velocity gunshot > 2,000 ft/sec
    Segmental fxs
    Segmental diaphyseal loss
    Farmyard injury

Mangled Extremity Severity Score *J Orthop Trauma 1994;8:81*
  Points and Category
    Skeletal/soft-tissue injury
      1 low energy (stab, simple fxs)
      2 medium energy (open or multiple fxs)
      3 high energy (crush)
      4 very high energy (above + gross contamination)
    Limb ischemia (category score doubles if > 6 hours)
      1 pulse reduced or absent with normal perfusion
      2 pulseless, paresthesias, diminished cap refill
      3 cool, paralyzed, insensate

Shock
  0 systolic blood pressure always > 90 mmHg
  1 transient hypotension
  2 persistent hypotension
Age (years)
  0 < 30
  1 30-50
  2 > 50
MESS score > 7 has high correlation with amputation

Compartment syndrome *OKU8-437, BJ255/281*
  Critical pressure > 30 mmHg
  Difference between DBP and compartment pressure < 30
    mmHg (may be more reliable)
  Suspect arterial injury if ABI < 0.90 ▶ arteriogram

Amputation *OKU7-128*
  Criteria for successful wound healing
    ABI $\geq$ 0.45 or absolute Doppler pressure 70 mmHg
    $TcpO_2 \geq$ 20-30 mmHg
    albumin $\geq$ 3.5 g/dl
    total lymphocyte count $\geq$ 1500
    toe pressure $\geq$ 30 mmHg

Pathologic fxs *OKU7-178, BJ392*
  Criteria for impending fx requiring ORIF
    > 2.5-3 cm lesion
    > 50% of cortex involved
    pain with weight bearing
    radiolucent lesion in the femoral neck involving 2/3
      diameter with associated pain

HAND

Open fx of the hand *RG736*
   Type I
      Clean, no systemic illness ▶ no abx
   Type II
      Contaminated, > 24 hrs delay in tx, systemic dz ▶
         cephazolin, and do not primarily close wounds
   Type III
      Greater than 2 cm wound length
      Crush component ▶ add aminoglycoside
      Bites or barnyard injury ▶ add PCN

Nailbed injury *G389*
   Traditional: if > 50% subungal hematoma ▶ consider removal
      nailplate and repair nailbed laceration; however, some
      studies show that trephination alone is adequate for
      hematomas up to 100% of the nail bed if the nail plate is
      intact and in place (*J Hand Surg 1999;24A:1166*, and *Am J
      Emerg Med 1991;9:209*)

Mallet finger *G192, RG677, BJ1240, HSU10*
   Tendinous mallet ▶ extension splinting
   Bony mallet, simple ▶ extension splinting
   Bony mallet, marked volar subluxation or > 30-50% articular
      surface involvement ▶ operative fixation

Phalangeal fx *G301, RG694, BJ1160, HSU6*
   Unstable spiral oblique fxs ▶ operate
   Condylar fxs ▶ operate
   Nondisplaced unicondylar fxs ▶ nonoperative treatment risky,
      need very close f/u
   Avulsion fxs at the base
      < 20-25% articular involvement ▶ splint for 2-3 weeks,
         then mobilize

> 2 mm displacement or instability ▶ open treatment

Tolerances

0-10° malrotation

1 mm step-off for intra-articular fxs

5-10° angulation in sagittal and coronal planes for shaft fxs

20° in sagittal plane for metaphyseal fxs

> 25-30° apex volar angulation (results in pseudoclawing)

Avoid immobilization for > 4 weeks for any phalangeal fxs

Metacarpal fx *G277, RG714, BJ1174, HSU29*

Tolerances – head

Noncommunited fxs with > 25% head involvement or > 1 mm articular step-off ▶ operate

Comminuted ▶ immobilize for 2 weeks at 70° flexion, then start aggressive ROM

Tolerances – neck

15° angulation for IF/LF

30-40° angulation for RF

50-60° angulation for SF, (even angulation of up to 70° has not been shown to cause loss of function)

Tolerances – shaft

Minimal displacement

No rotational deformity

5 mm shortening

10° coronal angulation

10° sagittal angulation for IF/LF

20° sagittal angulation for RF

30° sagittal angulation for SF

Tolerances – base

IF/LF/RF – controversial

SF CMC intra-articular fx-dislocation (Baby Bennett's) – inherently unstable ▶ CRPP

Thumb fx *G330, RG729, BJ1197, HSU47*
> Tolerances – shaft
>> 15-30° coronal angulation
>> 20-30° sagittal angulation
>
> Tolerances – extra-articular MC base
>> 20-30° angulation
>
> Bennet's fx (intra-articular fx at ulnar aspect of thumb base)
>> if < 15-20% of articular surface and > 1-2 mm disp ▶ CRPP
>> if > 25-30% of articular surface and > 1-2 mm disp ▶ ORIF
>
> Rolando's fx (Y-shaped intra-articular fx at thumb base)
>> ▶ ORIF, with possible pin supplementation or ex-fix
>> Restore joint congruity to < 2 mm

Thumb amputation *G1948, HSU57*
> Distal ¹/₃
>> ▶ soft tissue coverage
>
> Middle ¹/₃
>> Dist (retaining ¹/₂ of prox phal) ▶ deepen 1ˢᵗ web
>> Prox (near MP joint) ▶ MC lengthening, osteoplastic thumb reconstruction
>
> Proximal ¹/₃ (prox to neck of MC)
>> ▶ pollicization vs. toe transfer

Small joint arthrodesis *G454*
> MP: SF 40°, subtract 5° each digit radialward
> PIP: IF 40°, add 5° each digit ulnarward
> DIP: 0-5° for all; 5-10° supination may be helpful in IF/LF
> Thumb IP: 0-15°
> Thumb MP: 5-15° flexion with 10° pronation
> Thumb CMC: 40° palmar abduction, 20° radial abduction, and enough pronation for pulp to pulp contact with the fingers

DIP/PIP dorsal fx dislocation *G353, HSU10*

> < 40% articular surface involvement (stable) ▶ dorsal ext
> block splint vs. 7-14 days immobilization followed by
> buddy taping
>
> > 40% articular surface involvement ▶ consider volar plate
> arthroplasty vs dynamic ex-fix
>
> Single large fragment ▶ consider operative fixation

PIP dislocation *G345, RG688, BJ1244, HSU12*

> Lateral
> > < 20° laxity ▶ buddy tape 3 weeks
> > > 20° radio-ulnar laxity (complete collateral ligament injury)
> > ▶ buddy tape 3-6 weeks
> > Complete RCL rupture in IF ▶ consider repair in young
> > adult
>
> Dorsal (common)
> > Stable ▶ ext block splint or buddy tape
> > Irreducible (volar plate ruptured) ▶ operate
>
> Volar (rare)
> > Irreducible (often) or extensor lag > 30° ▶ operate
> > Fragment avulsed from dorsum with > 2 mm displacement
> > (central slip detachment) ▶ accurate open reduction

MP dislocation *RG706, HSU18*

> Locked dislocations ▶ operate
> Avulsion chip > 20% of articular surface and > 2 mm
> displacement ▶ operate

Skier's thumb (UCL rupture) *RG734, BJ1246, HSU49*

> > 30° more laxity than contralateral (tested in full extension
> and 30° flex) or > 35° laxity in full extension ▶ operate
> (HSU)

Thumb CMC dislocation *J Hand Surg 1996;21A:802-6*

> ▶ ligament reconstruction

Wrist

Tendon injury *G187*
  < 50% of extensor tendon lacerated ▶ do not repair
  < 60% of flexor tendon lacerated ▶ do not repair

WRIST

Wrist *RG756, OKU8-331, G538, HSU205*
  Normal load: 80% radius, 20% ulna
  Range of motion:
    Radial deviation: 20°
    Ulnar deviation: 40°
    Flexion/extension: 70° each
  Normal scaphoid axis (sagittal): 45° (range 30-60°) to capitate, lunate, and radius
  DISI: lunate > 10° extension (radiolunate angle)
  VISI: lunate > 15° flexion (radiolunate angle)
  S-L disruption indicated by S-L angle > 70° (80° is confirmatory), or R-S angle > 80°; C-L angle 20° is also suggestive
  S-L distance ≥ 3 mm is abnormal (normal = 1-2 mm)

Scaphoid fxs *RG784, OKU8-333, HSU161*
  Normal angles
    Lateral intrascaphoid angle: 30 ± 5°
    AP intrascaphoid angle: 40°
  Operative indications
    ≥ 1 mm stepoff
    ≥ 15° increase in intrascaphoid angulation
    > 60° S-L angle
    > 15° L-C angle
  Nonunion rate: 8-10%

Distal radius *RG856, G645, BJ1315*
  Normal measurements
    11-12° volar tilt

22° radial inclination
11-12 mm radial length (longitudinal length from tip of
   styloid to distal articular surface of ulna)
Tolerances (*JAAOS 1997;5:273*)
   Dorsal tilt: 15°
   Volar tilt: 20°
   Articular step-off: 2 mm
   Radial shortening: 5 mm
   Radial inclination: 15°
If > 15-20° initial dorsal angulation or > 4-5 mm impaction, fx
   is likely unstable
If > 25-30° initial fx angulation in sagittal plane, TFCC is
   probably disrupted
Fx at ulnar styloid base displaced > 3 mm indicates TFCC
   injury
Large styloid fragment > 3 mm displacement and/or gross
   DRUJ instability ▶ ORIF
4-5 mm intra-articular distal radius impaction ▶ bone graft
Chauffeur's fx (radial styloid) with > 3 mm displacement may
   have SLD
Barton's fx (intra-articular unstable fx subluxation of distal
   radius with volar or dorsal displacement) ▶ ORIF

FOREARM

Radius and ulnar shaft fxs *RG876*
   Operative indications
      All displaced both bone fxs and radius fxs
      Ulnar fxs > 10° angulation or > 50% displacement
      Compartment syndrome
      Galleazzi/Monteggia fxs
      Open fxs
   True X-ray views
      AP: bicipital tuberosity opposite radial styloid

Lat: ulnar styloid posterior, coronoid process anterior
Plate fixation tips
    Union rate after compression plating is > 96%
    Minimum fixation: 6 cortices on each side
    Lag screw fixation increases strength by up to 40%
Monteggia fxs – PIN most common nerve injured
    Bado classification
        I: ant dislocation of radial head (most common)
        II: posterolateral radial head dislocation
            A: ulnar fx at distal olecranon
            B: ulnar fx at metaphyseal/diaphyseal junction
            C: diaphyseal ulnar fx
            D: ulnar fx extends along proximal third to half of the
               ulna
        III: anterolateral/lateral radial head dislocation
        IV: ant radial head dislocation with radius fx
Galeazzi fxs – 3 times more common than Monteggia fxs
    Radiographic indications of disrupted DRUJ
        Fx at ulnar styloid base
        Widening of radial ulnar space on AP view
        Dislocation of ulna in relation to radius on lat view
        Radial shortening > 5 mm

ELBOW

Elbow *RG921, BJ1404, C3016, OKU8-307*
Articular cartilage surfaces of capitellum and trochlea project
    downward at 40° and at 4-8° valgus
Functional ROM = 30-130° ext-flex, 50° each supination and
    pronation
Up to 50% of proximal olecranon can be excised without
    creating instability (up to 80% in *RG939*)
Supracondylar fx
    Nondisplaced ▶ splint x 2 weeks

Displaced ▶ double plating

Medial epicondyle fxs (ossification center fuses at age 20)

    Operative indications

        Intraarticular fragment

        > 1 cm displacement

        Ulnar nerve palsy

    Otherwise ▶ splint in position of flexion and pronation for
10-14 days

Elbow dislocation

    If posterior dislocation is reduced and stable out to 30° of
flexion ▶ sling

    Acute recurrent dislocation ▶ hinged ex-fix

Coronoid process fxs

    Types

        I: tip avulsion

        II: fx involving < 50% of coronoid, not extending into
the base

        III: fx of > 50%, involving insertion of the brachialis and
ant band of MCL

    Instability or interference in ROM ▶ ORIF

Olecranon fxs

    Nondisplaced/stable (< 2 mm displacement with 0-90°
ROM) ▶ immobilize at 45-90° for 2-4 wks

    Displacement of ≥ 2 mm ▶ ORIF

Essex-Lopresti fxs—acute proximal translation of radius (radial
head fracture) with disruption of DRUJ (rupture of
interosseus membrane) ▶ do not excise radial head

Radial head fxs

    Radiocapitellar view: forearm neutral x-ray aimed 45°
cephalad

    Safe zone of radial head 90° centered on the point opposite
the lesser sigmoid notch in neutral rotation

    Classification and treatment

Type I: < 2 mm displacement and no limitation of
  sup/pron ▶ sling and active ROM; may need to
  immobilize for 2 weeks if > 1/3 of articular surface is
  involved
Type II: > 2 mm displacement, more than marginal lip;
  treatment controversial
  No limitation of ROM ▶ nonoperative
  Low demand patient ▶ consider head exision
  Essex-Lopresti or MCL rupture ▶ preserve or
    replace radial head
Type III: severe comminution ▶ excision or
  reconstruction/replacement of radial head (if elbow
  subluxated, with coronoid fx, Essex Lopresti, or MCL
  rupture)

HUMERUS

Humeral shaft fxs *RG977, BJ1481*
  > 90% union rate with nonoperative treatment
  Tolerances
    3 cm shortening (some sources say 5 cm)
    15° AP angulation
    15° varus/valgus angulation
    15° malrotation
  Operative indications
    Unacceptable alignment
    Spinal cord injury
    Lower extremity injury precluding weightbearing
    Multiple long bone fxs
    Pathologic fxs
    Floating elbow
    Bilateral fxs
    Vascular injury

Segmental fxs

Open fxs

Plating union rate: > 94%

Interlocked nails can be used if fx 2 cm distal to surgical neck or 3 cm proximal to olecranon fossa; nonunion rate up to 22%

Up to 18% of humeral shaft fxs have radial nerve injury, 90% will resolve in 3-4 months

Holstein-Lewis fx—oblique distal third fx commonly associated with radial nerve injury; however, some sources say middle third fxs are more commonly associated with radial nerve palsies

Indications for radial nerve exploration

Open fx

Penetrating injury

> 3½ months with no recovery

(Radial nerve palsy after manipulation not necessarily an operative indication *OKU7-268*)

Proximal Humerus Fxs *RG1007, BJ1512, OKU8-271*

6% associated with brachial plexus injury

Axillary nerve is the most commonly injured nerve

Musculocutaneous nerve enters coracobrachialis avg 5-6 cm from coracoid (range 3.1-8.2 cm)

X-ray series

1. AP of glenohumeral joint

2. Lateral in scapular plane

3. Axillary lateral

Morphology

Neck-shaft angle = 143° (range 134-166°)

Retroversion = 25° (range 26-31°)

Head offset = 3 mm posterior and 7 mm medial from center of humeral shaft

AVN rate = 13-34% with 4 part fxs, 3-13% with 3 part fxs

Main blood supply to humeral head: anterior humeral
circumflex artery

Head impaction fx

< 20% articular surface involved ▶ nonoperative

20-40% head involved ▶ McLaughlin procedure (transfer
lesser tuberosity), or rotational osteotomy

> 40% head involvement ▶ prosthetic replacement

Never split deltoid > 5 cm from edge of acromion to avoid
denervation

Tolerances

< 1 cm disp or < 45° angulation (unless otherwise noted)

The following fxs must have > 1 cm disp or > 45°
angulation to be classified as separate parts (0.5 cm disp
for greater tuberosity)

2 part surgical neck fxs ▶ closed reduction with or without
percutaneous pinning

Impacted fxs with > 45° angulation ▶ reduce (pin if
unstable)

2 part anatomic neck fxs ▶ early prosthetic replacement, or
open reduction if young

2 part greater tuberosity fxs > 5 mm disp ▶ ORIF, with
early passive ROM

2 part lesser tuberosity fxs—if small without decreased
ROM ▶ sling; if large with decreased IR ▶ ORIF

3 part fxs—if young and active ▶ ORIF; if osteoporotic ▶
prosthetic replacement

4 part fxs ▶ prosthetic replacement; consider attempt at
ORIF if good bone quality

SHOULDER GIRDLE

Glenoid fxs *OKU8-269, RG1090, BJ1631, DD989*

Glenoid normally faces anteriorly 45° (perpendicular to the
plane of scapular body)

Neck > 40° angulation or > 1-2 cm displacement ▶ ORIF

Intraarticular > 25% glenoid surface involved, > 5 mm steepoff ▶ ORIF

if comminuted, up to 25% of anterior lip can be excised and labrum reattached

Glenohumeral dislocation *RG1195, CH470*

80-90% redislocation rate after primary traumatic dislocation in teens

10-15% redislocation rate after primary traumatic dislocation age > 40 years

Anterior dislocation in 84%

Glenohumeral arthrodesis *OKU7-293*

Flexion: 20-30%

Abduction: 25-40%

Internal rotation: 25-30%

SLAP lesions *OKU8-260, OKUSpt190*

Type I: fraying with intact anchor ▶ debride

Type II: detachment of biceps anchor

Type III: bucket handle tear of superior labrum, biceps intact ▶ debride

Type IV: bucket handle tear of superior labrum including biceps anchor

If > 50% of the biceps tendon is torn in types II or IV ▶ biceps tenodesis, and stabilize labrum

Rotator cuff tears *OKU7-287*

Partial thickness RCTs with > 50% thickness of tendon torn ▶ repair

Massive tear > 5 cm or including ≥ 2 tendons: significant incidence of re-tear

Scapula fractures *RG1080, BJ1633, OKU8-269*
   High association with other injuries
   Scapular spine fx at base of acromion with > 5 mm disp ▶
      consider ORIF

Acromion *RG1094*
   Os acromiale: 2.7% of population, 60% bilateral
   X-ray views: include axillary lateral, supraspinatus outlet, and
      30° caudal tilt views
   Nondisplaced ▶ sling for 3 weeks
   Acromio-humeral space compromise ▶ ORIF

Coracoid *RG1095*
   get Stryker notch or 35° cephalic tilt view
   If isolated fx ▶ no specific tx
   Indications for surgery
      Associated with ≥ grade III AC separation
      Brachial plexus compression
      Obstruction of glenohumeral reduction
      Displaced fx with involvement of glenoid fossa

Scapulothoracic dissociation *RG1106*
   On AP Radiograph: if medial border of scapula to thoracic
      spine is > 1.5x the contralateral side

AC joint injuries *RG1215*
   Injury classification
      Type I: sprain AC ligament ▶ ice x 12 hours then ROM
      Type II: AC joint disruption, CC ligament sprain with slight
         widening and vertical separation ▶ ice x 12 hours, sling,
         then gentle ROM after 1 week, no heavy lifting and no
         contact sports for 8-12 weeks
      Type III: CC interspace 25-100% more than normal
         shoulder

Operative indications
    Heavy laborers
    Concomitant brachial plexus injury
    Overhand athlete's dominant arm
Type IV: posterior dislocation ▶ operate
Type V: 100-300% CC space ▶ operate
Type VI: inferior clavicular dislocation ▶ operate

Floating shoulder *RG1061*
    Combined fx of clavicle and glenoid neck
    Operative indications
        Medial glenoid displacement > 3 cm
        Clavicle fx displacement meets indication for ORIF
        Multiple trauma with need for upper ext wt bearing for
            rehab
        > 40° of abnormal glenoid version

Clavicle *RG1046, BJ1633, OKU8-267*
    3% risk of pneumothorax with clavicle fx
    Coracoid to clavicle average distance = 1.3 cm
    X-rays: obtain cephalic tilt view
    AP/lat trauma series helpful for distal 1/3 fxs
    Classification
        Group I: middle 1/3—80% of clavicle fxs
        Group II: distal 1/3—12-15% of clavicle fxs
            Type I: interligamentous (most common)
            Type IIa: conoid and trapezoid on distal fragment
            Type IIb: trapezoid on distal fragment, conoid ruptured
            Type III: distal intraarticular fx
            Type IV: pseudodislcation (children < 16 y/o)
            Type V: comminuted, neither of the major fragments
                have ligamentous support
        Group III: proximal 1/3—5-8% of clavicle fxs

Nonunion rate: 1-4% overall

    Distal 1/3 more prone, but still 75-85% of nonunions occur in middle 1/3 (30% atrophic, 70% hypertrophic)

Operative indications for midshaft fxs

    Absolute

        Shortening ≥ 20 mm

        Open injury

        Impending skin disruption with irreducible fx

        Vascular compromise

        Progressive neurologic loss

        Displaced pathologic fx assc with trapezial paralysis

        Scapulothoracic dissociation

    Relative

        Displacement > 20 mm

        Neurologic disorder (Parkinson's, seizure, head injury)

        Multiple trauma

        Expected prolonged recumbency

        Floating shoulder

        Ipsilateral upper extremity fx

        Bilateral fxs

<u>Sternoclavicular joint *RG1273, DD946*</u>

    X-ray: serendipity view—40° cephalic tilt AP

    Sprain without dislocation ▶ ice

    Anterior dislocation (most common) ▶ closed reduction

        If stable ▶ figure-8 brace

        If unstable ▶ sling for 7 days, then ROM

    Posterior dislocation ▶ closed vs. open reduction; consider pre-op CT or angiogram

SPINE

C-spine *RG1328, BJ777*

    Checklist for the Diagnosis of Clinical Instability

        Points: Element

            2: anterior elements destroyed or unable to function

            2: posterior elements destroyed or unable to function

            2: relative sagittal plane translation > 3.5 mm

            2: relative sagittal plane rotation > 11°

            2: posterior stretch test

            2: cord injury

            1: root injury

            1: abnormal disc narrowing

            1: congenital spinal stenosis

            1: dangerous loading anticipated

        Clinical instability if > 5 points

    Radiography

        Powers ratio (atlanto-occipital dissociation) basion to posterior arch of atlas/opisthion to anterior arch of atlas, if > 1.0 suspect injury

        Dens basion interval should be < 12 mm

        Space available for the cord should be > 13 mm

        Atlanto-dens interval in adult is normally < 3 mm

        odontoid to C1 medial border (lateral atlanto-dental space) seen on AP view should be equal bilaterally, but a discrepancy of 2 mm or greater can be seen in patients without pathology

        Retropharyngeal soft tissue

            Normal < 6 mm at C2

            Normal < 18 mm at C6

Jefferson's fx—symmetric axial compression, fracturing ring of C1 in several locations (widening of lateral masses), > 8.0 mm total overhang of C1 on C2 or atlanto-dens interval > 4 mm on lateral view indicates transverse ligament rupture (neurologic injury rarely associated)

Treatment based on stability

If stable posterior arch fx or nondisplaced fxs of the anterior and posterior portion of the ring ▶ cervical orthosis

Combined lateral mass overhang 2-7 mm, patients with 3-4 fxs of the C1 ring, or asymmetric lat mass fxs ▶ halo vest x 3 m

Halo orthosis: most stable form of external immobilization; neck motion 4% f/e, 4% lat bending, 1% rotation

Combined lat mass overhang > 7 mm (transverse lig rupture) ▶ internal fixation/fusion C1-2 vs 4-6 wks traction, then 2 months halo vest until healing of C1 ring, then fuse if ADI > 4 mm (adults) or > 5 mm (children) on flexion/extension views or if symptomatic

Consider fusion after initial reduction with traction if massively unstable

Simple rotation and lateral bending can give up to 4 mm overhang on open-mouth odontoid view, and congenital anomalies may produce 1-2 mm offset

Hangman's fxs *OKU7-598, RG1335, BJ795*

Traumatic spondylolisthesis of the axis (bilateral pars or articular facet fxs); second most common axis injury after odontoid fxs

30% incident of concomitant c-spine fxs

Classification and treatment
Type I: 29%
Nondisplaced; no angulation; translation < 3 mm C2 on
C3; C2-3 disc intact (stable); ► c-collar x 6 wks
Type II: 56%
Significant angulation and ≥ 3 mm translation; usually
has associated compression fx of C3 (unstable); ►
reduction and halo for at least 6 wks
Type IIA: 6%
Severe angulation; no translation; disruption of PLL
(unstable); ► halo in extension (gets worse with
traction)
Type III: 9%
Severe angulation and translation; unilateral or bilateral
facet dislocation of C2-3; ► open reduction and
posterior fusion of C1-2

AA rotatory subluxation *RG1333, BJ786*

Atlanto-axial joint normally allows 40° motion to each side
With an intact transverse ligament, complete bilateral
dislocation of the articular processes can occur at ~65° of
AA rotation, with significant narrowing of the spinal canal
and vertebral artery compromise. Or with transverse
ligament deficiency, complete unilateral dislocation can
occur at 45° rotation with similar consequences. Diagnosis
requires persistent asymmetry of the odontoid and its
relationship to the articular masses on open mouth views
with the head rotated 15° to each side.
Classification
Type I: ADI < 3 mm, transverse ligament intact
Type II: ADI 3-5 mm, transverse ligament insufficient
Type III: ADI > 5 mm, failure of alar ligaments
Type IV: complete posterior dislocation of the atlas (dens
usually deficient, rare)

Type V: frank rotatory dislocation (extremely rare)

Treatment varies from ROM with supine cervical halter traction followed by cervical orthosis, to reduction with Gardner-Wells traction followed by halo immobilization. AA fusion is occasionally indicated for persistent instability.

Fxs of the odontoid process *RG1335, BJ789, OKU7-597*

Type I: 5%

Oblique fxs of upper portion (alar lig avulsion) ► cervical orthosis

If unstable (AO dissociation) ► cervical fusion

Type II: 60%

Most common fx of upper c-spine associated with primary neurological injury (18-25% incidence)

Fx at the dens-central body of axis junction (risk for nonunion 36%)

Surgical indications for C1-2 fusion

Absolute

> 5-6 mm disp

> 60 y/o

Failure of previous reduction

Nonunion

Relative

Presenting > 2-3 weeks post injury

Angulation > 10°

Polytrauma

Type III: 30%

Fx line extends into cancellous bone of the body of axis ► halo x 2 months

Lat mass fxs *BJ795*

Potentially unstable; however, if no significant fx of the facet complexes and < 20% compression of the lat mass ► two-poster brace with close follow-up

Solumedrol protocol (controversial) *NASCIS III Trial. JAMA 1997;
227:1597-1604*
  If < 3 hrs ▶ 30 mg/kg over 15 min then 5.4 mg/kg x 23 hrs
  If 3-8 hrs ▶ same x 48 hrs
  If > 8 hrs ▶ nothing
  Remember H2 blocker

Cervical spinal canal stenosis *OKU7-614*
  Pavlov's ratio: sagittal canal diameter/sagittal vertebral body
    diameter
    A ratio of 0.8 or less defines a narrow cervical canal
  Normal AP diameter = 13-17 mm
  10 mm = absolute stenosis
  < 7 mm = critical stenosis
  Compression ratio (ratio of the smallest sagittal cord diameter
    to the largest transverse cord diameter at the same level)
    If < 0.4 = poor prognosis
    Expanding ratio to > 0.4 correlates with clinical recovery

Rheumatoid arthritis *OKU7-691*
  Anterior atlanto-dens interval normal < 3 mm
  Posterior atlanto-dens interval
    Normal > 14 mm; if > 14 mm, then 94% without
      neurological deficit
    If ≤ 14 mm ▶ MRI
  Consider fusion if MRI shows the following
    Cervicomedullary angle < 135°
    Cord diameter ≤ 6 mm
    Space available for the cord < 13 mm

Throacolumbar spine parameters *RG1405*
  40% of C-spine fractures and 15-20% of T-L spine fxs have
    neurologic injury
  Spinal cord 35% of canal at atlas, 50% of canal in lower C-
    spine and T-L spine

Cord ends at caudal end of L1 vertebral body
Denis 3 column concept
    Anterior column: ALL, anterior 2/3 of vertebral body
    Middle column: posterior 1/3 of vertebral body and PLL
    Posterior column: bony arch, pedicles, facets, laminae,
        posterior ligaments

Thoracolumbar spine injuries *OKU7-603,OKUSpine128, RG1450,*
BJ875
Compression fxs: ant column only, no mid or post column
    distraction
    If < 40% to 50% loss of height or < 20° to 30° kyphosis ▶
        hyperextension brace; occasionally PSIF recommended
        (progressive deformity or neuro compromise)
    If > 40% to 50% loss of height or > 20° to 30° kyphosis ▶
        consider PSIF
    Osteoporotic compression fxs
        ▶ CT if at lordotic L-spine (mid column involvement
          more common)
        ▶ lab w/u especially if male
        Pain minimal ▶ Jewett brace
        Chronic pain ▶ consider vertebroplasty/kyphoplasty
Simple posterior column injuries
    Types
        Spinous process fxs
        Transverse process fxs
        Isolated laminar fxs
        Articular process fxs
    ▶ symptomatic treatment
Isolated pars interarticularis fxs ▶ TLSO
Burst fxs: ant/mid column ± post column
    Indications for PSIF (unstable burst)
        > 50% loss of height
        > 20° kyphotic deformity

> 10° scoliosis
> 50% canal compromise
posterior element injury
incomplete neurologic deficit associated with canal
    compromise

Fx-dislocation: disruption of all 3 columns by compression
    and/or rotation, shear (translational injuries), neuro deficit
    common ▶ operative management

Chance fx: all columns fail in distraction (no translation)
    Bony elements only ▶ total contact TLSO or
        hyperextension cast x 3 months
    If line of force involves ligaments/disc space ▶ surgical
        stabilization

Flexion-distraction: ant column compression, mid/post column
    distraction
    Instability if
        ≥ 20° kyphosis
        > 33 mm interspinous distance on AP view
    Impending if
        > 12° kyphosis
        > 20 mm interspinous distance
    ▶ total contact TLSO or hyperextension cast x 3 months
4-5% have additional noncontiguous spine fxs

Bracing for "stable" fxs *BJ894, OKUSpine169, JAAOS*
1995;3:353, Orthop Rev 1992;21:753

Stable fractures: criteria
    No transient or persistent neurologic injury
    Acceptable alignment
    At least one column intact
    No significant ligamentous rupture

Bracing range for stable fxs
    Aspen collar: C1-C7
    Minerva: C1-T8
    Jewett: T6-L3
    CTLSO: C1-L3 (fxs present both above T6 and below T8)
    TLSO: T6-L3
    HTLSO: T6-sacrum

Duration of bracing treatment
    Fxs above T7 ▶ 8-12 weeks
    Fxs below T7 ▶ 12-16 weeks
    L4 and below ▶ include single leg immobilization for 6-12
        weeks

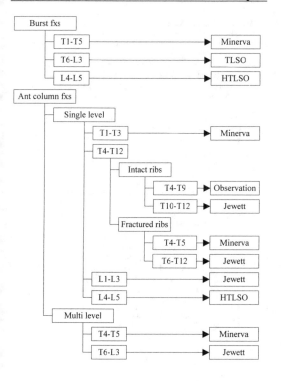

Spine

GSW to spine *BJ983, RG1317*

   If progressive neuro deficit with demonstrable neural
      compression from bullet, fx fragments, or hematoma ▶
      operate

   If incomplete neurologic injury ▶ decompress

   Uncontaminated wound ▶ 3 days IV abx

   Perforated viscus ▶ general surgery repair of viscus and local
      debridement (small bowel perforations do not need spinal
      debridement); then broad spectrum IV abx for 1-2 weeks

   If military weapon ▶ serial debridements

   CSF leak or fistula ▶ dural repair

   Evaluate stability

      C-spine: 36% of head weight is supported through the
         anterior vertebral bodies and 32% is supported by each
         of the posterolateral columns

      T and L spine: apply Denis 3 column concept

         If none of these 3 columns is disrupted ▶ no
            immobilization

         If one column disrupted ▶ rigid cervical collar for C-
            spine, nothing for T and L spine

         If two or three columns disrupted ▶ halo vest for C-
            spine, TLSO for T and L spines

         If columns are not significantly disrupted,
            immobilization is rarely indicated, unless progressive
            deformity is documented on upright films

      In contrast to closed injuries, GSWs rarely require
         operations for purposes of stability

Herniated disk, DDD *OKU7-634*

   Surgical indications

      Urgent

         Cauda equina syndrome

         Progressive neuro deficit

Elective
Predominately leg pain > 6 weeks
Failure of reasonable conservative treatment
Nerve root tension sign (+SLR)
Radiographic evidence (MRI/CT myelogram)
Dynamic criteria for degenerative segmental instability
Translation > 4 mm and/or 10° angular difference on lateral
flex/ext radiographs
Rotatory hypermobility > 15° on lat view
Disk wedging > 5° on AP view
Lateral translation > 3 mm
Removal of > 50% of both facets or 100% of one facet can
cause instability

Lumbar spinal stenosis *BD1537*
Normal canal: ≥ 12 mm
Canal stenosis: ≤ 10 mm AP diameter
Lateral recess stenosis: < 2 mm

Metastatic disease of the spine *BJ405, OKUSpine427*
Asymptomatic
No deformity or canal compromise ▶
chemotherapy/hormonal therapy
Significant structural involvement (> 50% body destruction)
▶ radiation if sensitive
Symptomatic – pain
< 50% body destruction and no canal compromise ▶
radiation if sensitive
> 50% body destruction or instability or canal compromise
▶ surgery
Symptomatic – neurologic deficit
≥ 10% of patients with neurologic deficit from metastatic
disease have at least 2 areas of compression
▶ surgery

Relative contraindications to surgery
Multiple nonadjacent levels of canal compromise
Poor bone quality
Life expectancy < 3 months
Complete paraplegia > 2 days

Adult scoliosis *OKU7-654, OKUSpine378*
If < 30°, unlikely to progress
If thoracic curve > 60° or lumbar curve > 50°, expect 1-2°
progression/year
Surgical indications
Documented progression of thoracic curves > 50-60°
Double major curves > 60°
Lumbar curves > 50°
Curves > 50° with pain unresponsive to nonsurgical
measures
Thoracic curves > 80-90° with diminished pulmonary
fuction
Lumbar curves with rotatory subluxations causing axial pain
or spinal stenosis
Indications for circumferential fusion
Large curves > 60°
Any kyphotic component to lumbar region
Osteoporosis
Fusion to sacrum

Spondylolisthesis *OKUSpine103*
3-6% of population
Diagnosis
Lateral x-ray
SPECT scan
CT with thin cuts
Grades of slip
1: 1-25%

2: 26-50%
3: 51-75%
4: 76-100%
5: > 100% (spondyloptosis)

Treatment
Rest, brace, stretching, strengthening
Consider fusion if ≥ grade 3

PELVIS AND ACETABULUM

Pelvis *RG1487, BJ1052, C2962, OKU8-387*
Pubic diastasis > 2.0-2.5 cm ▶ ex-fix vs ORIF
> 1 cm displacement at SI joint or leg length discrepancy > 1
    cm indicates instability
Throckmorton sign: positive if angle of the dangle is > 0°
    pointing toward the lesion (male patients only)
    If angle of the dangle > 90° ▶ use extreme caution
Injury classification (Young system)
    LC: transverse fracture of pubic rami, ipsilateral or
        contralateral to posterior injury
        I: sacral compression on side of impact
        II: crescent (iliac wing) fracture on side of impact
        III: LC-1 or LC-II injury on side of impact; contralateral
            open-book (APC) injury
    APC: symphyseal diastasis or longitudinal rami fxs
        I: slight widening of pubic symphysis (< 2.5 cm) or ant
            SI joint; stretched but intact ant SI, sacrotuberous,
            and sacrospinous ligaments; intact post SI ligaments
            ▶ nonoperative tx
        II: widened ant SI joint; disrupted anterior SI,
            sacrotuberous, and sacrospinous ligaments; intact
            posterior SI ligaments ▶ ant fixation ± post fixation

III: complete SI joint disruption, including sacrotuberous
and sacrospinous ligaments; disrupted posterior SI
ligaments ▶ post fixation ± ant fixation; after
fixation of post, if residual gap or fx disp > 2 cm ant
or instability on exam requires ant fixation

VS: symphyseal diastasis or vertical displacement anteriorly
and posteriorly; usually through the SI joint (> 1 cm
superior translation), occasionally through the iliac wing
or sacrum

CM: combination of other injury patterns, LC/VS being the
most common

Acetabulum *RG1531, BJ1109, OKU8-392*

Criteria for nonoperative treatment

Severe osteoporosis

> 10 mm intact dome on CT (intact 45° arc medially from
vertical line drawn through the center of the femoral
head; fx will cross weight bearing dome if roof arc < 45°)

< 2-3 mm displacement

Congruent acetabulum in a both column fx

< 50% of posterior wall fx with a stable reduction (< 40%
by CT measurements)

Letournel and Judet classifications, with surgical approach

Posterior wall ▶ Kocher-Langenbeck

Posterior column ▶ Kocher-Langenbeck

Anterior wall ▶ ilioinguinal

Anterior column ▶ ilioinguinal, EIF

Transverse ▶ Kocher-Langenbeck

Posterior column-posterior wall ▶ Kocher-Langenbeck

Transverse and posterior wall ▶ Kocher-Langenbeck and
EIF

T-shaped ▶ Kocher-Langenbeck, EIF

Anterior-posterior hemitransverse ▶ ilioinguinal

Both column ▶ ilioinguinal, EIF

Hip arthroplasty *C315, CH2769, OKUHKR75*
    Acetabular component position
        10-20° anteversion
        45° inclination
    Tests for stability
        > 40° ER in extension
        > 45° IR in 90° flexion and neutral abduction
    Contraindications
        Relative
            Neuropathic arthropathy
            Abductor insufficiency
            Rabidly progressive neurologic disease
        Absolute
            Active infection
                Usefulness of intraop frozen section for infected THA,
                    sensitivity 100%, specificity 96%; criteria: ≥ 5
                    PMN/HPF; gold standard = intraop culture
            Unstable medical illness

Position for hip arthrodesis *C186, CH2843, OKU8-415*
    20-30° flexion
    0-5° adduction
    0-15° ER

Femoral head osteonecrosis *OKU8-415, C373, OKUHKR132,*
    JBJS 1996;78A:1032
    50% of atraumatic ON is bilateral
    Ficat stages
        0: asymptomatic with MRI changes only ▶ core
        decompression
        I: no radiographic signs, symptomatic, with early changes
        on MRI ▶ core decompression

II: porosis, sclerosis or cysts, crescent sign appears late ▶
    vascularized strut graft/core decompression

III: femoral head collapse (joint space nl) ▶
    hemiarthroplasty (or resurfacing)

IV: acetabular and femoral head involvement (arthritis) ▶
    THA

Indications for osteotomy

    < 45 y/o

    painful hip (Ficat I, II, or early III)

    20° arc of intact lateral head

    < 200° combined arc involvement on AP/lat

    no continued use of high dose steroids

    < 30% femoral head involvement

Femoral head fxs *RG1553, OKU7-408*

Pipkin classification

    I: fx caudad to fovea ▶ reduction to 2-3 mm vs excision

    II: fx cephalad to fovea ▶ reduction to 1-2 mm

    III: associated fx of femoral neck with type I or II (50%
    AVN rate) ▶ treat each component as separate injury

    IV: associated fx of acetabulum with type I, II, or III ▶ treat
    each component as separate injury

Femoral neck fxs *RG1586, BJ1700, C2908, OKU7-410*

Normal anatomy

    Antcversion 13 ± 7° (may approach 30° in Asian population)

    Neck-shaft angle in females: 133 ± 7°

    Neck-shaft angle in males: 129 ± 7°

    Neck-shaft angle decreases to 125° at age 70

Garden classification

    I: incomplete or impacted

    II: complete fx without displacement

    III: complete fx with partial displacement

    IV: complete fx with total displacement

Garden's index of acceptable reduction

Central axis of compressive trabeculae normally forms 160°
angle with the shaft on AP view, should be 160-180°
after reduction; on lateral view, should be < 10-20°
angulation

Displaced femoral neck fxs

< 65 y/o, no chronic dz ▶ immediate reduction (to ≤ 15°
valgus and < 10° post angulation) and fixation with
multiple pins/screws

65-75 with good bone density and high level of function ▶
ORIF

< 75 y/o with chronic dz ▶ hemiarthroplasty

> 75 y/o ▶ prosthetic replacement (hemiarthroplasty or
THA)

Pre-existing DJD ▶ THA

limited life expectancy ▶ hemiarthroplasty

Complications

Nondisplaced fxs

< 8-18% AVN rate

< 5% nonunion rate

10-27% disimpaction rate without fixation

Displaced fxs

15-33% AVN rate

10-30% nonunion rate

1/3 of hips with AVN require reoperation

3/4 of hips with nonunion require reoperation

Greater trochanteric fxs *RG1661*

If no comminution and > 1 cm displaced ▶ consider ORIF
(tension band wiring)

Intertrochanteric fxs *RG1645*

Nondisplaced/displaced ▶ ORIF vs intramedullary device

Reverse obliquity ▶ 95° blade plate vs intramedullary device
Nonambulatory ▶ may treat nonoperatively

FEMUR

Femoral shaft fxs *RG1685, BJ1879, OKU8-425*
  Winquist classification
    Type I: minimal or no comminution
    Type II: comminution involving < 50% of cortical diameter
    Type III: comminution of 50-100% of cortical diameter
    Type IV: segmental comminution
  Indications for prophylactic nailing (metastasis)
    1. Width of metastasis/width of bone > 0.6
    2. Axial cortical destruction > 30 mm
    3. Cortical destruction > 50% circumference of the shaft
  Tolerances
    5-10° varus
    10-15 mm shortening
    15° rotational malalignment
  Fxs occurring 6-8 cm proximal to distal articular surface and
    distal to lesser trochanter ▶ may be managed with a
    standard IMR
  Any butterfly fragments > 2 cm from fx site do not contribute
    to healing
  Retrograde femoral nailing
    Indications
      Multi-trauma
      Ipsilateral femoral neck/shaft fx
      Pulmonary/abdominal/pelvic injuries
      Obese patients
      Pregnancy
    Relative indications
      Ipsilateral acetabular fx
      Femoral shaft fx with ipsilateral arterial injury

Floating knee
Ipsilateral through-knee amputation
Ipsilateral in situ hip prosthesis

Supracondylar femur fxs *RG1738, BJ1957*
Tolerances
5-7° varus/valgus malalignment
7-10° AP malalignment (as seen on lat x-ray)
10-15 mm shortening
2 mm articular stepoff
Tolerances for periprosthetic knee fxs (if bone prosthetic
interface OK)
5 mm translation
5-10° angulation
10° rotation
1 cm shortening

Patellar fxs *RG1789, OKU8-433, BJ2013*
Tolerances
3 mm gap
2 mm stepoff
Must document intact extensor mechanism for nonoperative
tx

Patellar height *RG1867, DD1851*
Blackburne-Peel index A/B < 1.0 (nl = 0.8)
A = anterior plateau to inferior articular surface of patella
B = articular surface length of patella
Insall-Salvati index LT/LP < 1.02 (nl = 1.0) at 30° knee flexion

Chondromalacia *OKUSpt24, DD1881*
Outerbridge classification
Grade I: softening
Grade II: fragmentation and fissuring

Grade III: fibrillation (crabmeat appearance)

Grade IV: subchondral bone

Defects > 2 cm^2 rarely heal

Treatment—variable depending on anatomic location and size of lesion

Femoral condyle

< 2 cm^2 ▶ drilling/debridement; osteochondral plug repair, autologous chondrocyte implant for treatment of clinical failure

> 2 cm^2 ▶ osteochondral plug repair or autologous chondrocyte implant (best used on femoral condyles, not recommended for tibia); consider drilling/debridement for less active patients

Patella

Similar algorithm as femoral condyle after alignment is corrected

Tibial plateau

Autologous chondrocyte implant and mosaicplasty not recommended

Degenerative knee joint *OKUHKR258,302, C243, CH2860*

Unicompartmental arthroplasty (*OKU8-459*)

Indications and requirements

Unicompartmental DJD

Age ≥ 60 years

Weight < 180 lbs

Not heavy laborer

Knee flexion arc ≥ 90° with < 5° flexion contracture

Angular deformity < 10°

Intact ACL

Noninflammatory arthritis

High tibial osteotomy

Indications and requirements

Age < 60-65 years

Isolated medial compartment DJD
10-15° varus deformity when weightbearing
Arc of motion ≥ 90° with < 15° flexion contracture
Contraindications
Inflammatory arthritis
Lateral tibial subluxation > 1 cm
Medial compartment bone loss > 2-3 mm
Loss of lateral compartment joint space
Ligamentous instability
Goal
5-7° valgus overcorrection
Distal femoral osteotomy
Indications and requirements
Younger patients
Isolated lateral compartment DJD
Valgus deformity < 15°
Valgus joint line tilt > 10°
Arc of motion ≥ 90° with < 10° flexion contracture
Goal
Correct tibiofemoral angle to 4-6° valgus
Knee arthrodesis—optimal position
5-7° valgus
10° ER
0-15° flexion

Meniscal tears *RG1878, BJ2061, DD1675*
Classification
Grade I: small disruption of homogenous signal
Grade II: more pronounced but does not extend to surface
Grade III: tear with extension to either surface
Peripheral tear and < 1 cm, partial thickness or displaces < 3 mm ► no treatment indicated
Tear in outer 1/3 (< 4 mm outer rim width) ► repair
Tear in inner 2/3 ► partial meniscectomy

Femur

ACL injury *OKUSpt307*

Laxity > 3 mm side to side difference = ACL rupture
Improved healing rates of meniscal repair when combined with reconstruction
Timing of surgery
Wait until nontender nonswollen knee with full ROM
Patellar tendon autograft is the "gold standard"
Consider conservative tx in older patients willing to modify lifestyle

PCL injury *OKUSpt317, DD1978, 2090*

> 10° increased ER at 90° knee flexion = PCL injury
Avulsion fx at site of PCL tibial insertion with > 5 mm disp ► operate
60% of PCL tears are associated with PLC injuries
If grade III laxity (> 10 mm) after rehab ► consider reconstruction

Posterolateral corner injury *OKU8-448*

> 10° increased ER at 30° knee flexion
15% have peroneal n. injury with grade III LCL injury
Acute
Grade I and II ► nonsurgical
Grade III ► repair within 1-2 weeks
Chronic
Grade III ► reconstruction
Grade III with varus deformity ► opening wedge medial proximal tibial osteotomy with reconstruction

MCL injury *OKU7-492*

Test at 30° flexion
Classification
Grade I: 1-5 mm opening
Grade II: 6-10 mm opening
Grade III: ≥ 11 mm opening

Treatment
> Grades I, II, III ▶ symptomatic treatment with crutches until no limp, then d/c crutches; benefits from the use of braces during initial healing is inconclusive
>
> Continued grade III instability after 3-4 weeks of rehab ▶ may require surgical reconstruction

TIBIA AND FIBULA

Tibial plateau fxs *RG1807, OKU7-480, BJ2074*
> Classification (Schatzker)
>> I: lateral plateau split
>> II: lateral plateau split depression
>> III: isolated lateral depression
>> IV: medial plateau fx
>> V: bicondylar plateau fx
>> VI: bicondylar fx with metaphyseal diaphyseal dissociation
>
> Tolerances
>> < 5-10° varus/valgus instability
>> < 1.5-3.0 mm joint line incongruity
>
> Wire placement should be ≥ 15 mm from joint to avoid septic knee

Tibia fxs *OKU8-438, BJ2131*
> Tolerances
>> 5° varus/valgus angulation
>> 5° AP angulation
>> 15° IR
>> 20° ER
>> 12-20 mm shortening
>> 50% displacement
>
> If > 15 mm initial shortening, nontransverse fx ▶ IMR
>> Cast bracing should not be used if > 15 mm initial shortening

Intact fibula: relative contraindication to closed treatment
(*CORR 1995;315:8*)
Requirements for IMR
Minimal canal diameter = 8 mm
Fx zone 5 cm below knee
Fx zone 1-5 cm above ankle depending on implant design
Static lock all fxs with > 25% cortical diameter comminution

ANKLE

Ankle *RG2002, OKU7-547, OKUFA188*
10° DF and 20° PF needed for normal walking
Normal radiographic measurements on mortise view
Tibiofibular line should be continuous
Talar tilt normal angle < 5°
Talar tilt > 10-15° or 2x uninjured side with stress is
abnormal
Superior clear space from med to lat should vary ≤ 2 mm
Talocrural angle 83 ± 4°
Weber classification for ankle fractures
A: below level of the plafond
B: at the level of the plafond
C: above the level of the plafond

Isolated lateral malleolus fxs *OKUFA189, OKU7-206*
Tolerances
3 mm displacement (supination-external rotation II)
2-5° side-to-side difference in talocrural angle

Isolated medial malleolus fxs *OKUFA190*
Nondisplaced fxs ▶ NWB cast immobilization 4-6 weeks
Displaced fxs ▶ ORIF

Medial and lateral injuries *RG2027, OKUFA190, OKUT206*
> 1 mm lateral talar displacement ► anatomic fixation of lateral malleolus (ORIF of medial malleolus if displaced)

If medial clear space is > 2 mm more than normal after reduction of fibula or if reduction is blocked (> 2 mm talar shift) ► explore medial side

Posterior malleolus: if > 25% articular and > 2mm articular displacement ► ORIF

Syndesmotic injury *OKU7-549, BJ2344, C2730, OKUFA188, OKUT208, Foot Ankle Int 1994;15:407, JAAOS 1997;5:172*
Indications for fixation
> 2 mm lateral talar shift

Tib-fib clear space ≥ 6 mm (separation of fibular from lateral border of tibial notch on mortise x-ray measured 1 cm above joint line)

Medial clear space > 4 mm or > 2.5 mm increase with ER stress view

Tib/fib overlap < 1 mm on mortise view

Positive stress test

Syndesmotic injuries extending < 3.5 cm from plafond do not need syndesmotic screw with anatomic fibular fixation (even with deltoid ligament rupture), unless stress test is positive

Syndesmotic fixation may not be necessary if rigid bimalleolar fixation is obtained and fibula fx is within 15 cm of the tibiotalar joint, unless stress test is positive

Syndesmotic screw fixation should be left in place for at least 12 weeks

Chronic ligamentous instability of the ankle *OKU7-557*
Talar tilt 3-5° > contralateral limb or absolute value > 9°

10 mm anterior drawer or 3 mm greater than opposite side ► consider operative treatment

Ankle arthrodesis *C155, OKUFA284*
  0-5° valgus
  0° DF/PF
  5-10° ER
  slight posterior displacement of the talus

FOOT

Talar neck fxs *RG2094, OKU7-553, BJ2379, OKUFA204*
  Classification
    Type I: nondisplaced vertical fx (absolutely no
        displacement), 10% osteonecrosis rate (0-13%) ▶ NWB
        cast in slight PF x 4 wks, then SLWC x 8 wks
    Type II: displaced fx with subluxation/dislocation of the
        subtalar joint, 40% osteonecrosis rate (20-50%) ▶
        emergency anatomic ORIF
    Type III: displaced fx with dislocation of body from subtalar
        and ankle joints, 90% osteonecrosis rate (50-100%) ▶
        emergency anatomic ORIF
    Type IV: a type III fx with talar head dislocation, 100%
        osteonecrosis rate ▶ emergency anatomic ORIF
  3/5 of talus is covered by articular cartilage
  > 5 mm medial disp of calcaneus on the talus indicates excess
      subtalar joint laxity
  Hawkin's sign: best x-ray indication of viability of talar body,
      time to recognize AVN is 6-8 wks post fx. AP x-ray of
      ankle reveals presence or absence of subchondral osteopenia
      in talar dome. Subchondral osteopenia (Hawkin's sign)
      excludes the dx of AVN.

Osteochondral talus fxs *RWB1186, OKUFA40, 211*
  Classification (modified Berndt-Harty)
    Stage I: confined to trabecular compression, only seen on
        MRI
    Stage II: incomplete separation of osteochondral fragment

Stage IIa: if a subchondral cyst is present
Stage III: fragment completely detached but undisplaced
Stage IV: displaced fragment
Treatment
Stages I and II ▶ 6 wks NWB immobilization
Stages III, IV, and failed stages I and II ▶ arthroscopic
debridement, drilling, or mosaicplasty (lesions > 10 mm)

Calcaneus *RG2133, OKUFA216*
Radiography
AP (dorsoplantar), lateral, axial (Harris) views
CT – coronal, axial, and sagittal views
Optional
Brodens (for posterior facet) – AP with foot internally
rotated 45°, tube tilted cephalad at 40°, 30°, 20°, and
10°
Lateral oblique view (for anterior process avulsion fxs) –
45° caudad lateral
Normal Bohler's tuber joint angle = 25-40°
Normal crucial angle of Gissane = 135 ± 10°
80-90% of fxs result from a fall
5-9% bilateral
10% associated with spinal compression fxs
Tongue type: one large posterior/superior and lateral
fragment
Joint depression type: more common, fx line deviates
dorsally exiting just posterior to the articular facet
Sanders classification (based on CT)
Type I: all nondisplaced articular fxs ▶ nonoperative
Type II: displaced 2 part fxs of the posterior fact ▶
ORIF if soft tissue allows
Type III: displaced fxs with 3 articular fragments, the
central fragment frequently being depressed ▶ ORIF
if soft tissue allows

Type IV: displaced fxs with 4 or more articular
fragments with high comminution ▶ nonoperative
treatment

Anterior process displaced fxs and > 1 cm in size ▶ ORIF

Avulsion fxs of the posterior tuberosity
Nondisplaced ▶ plantar flexion cast 3-4 wks, then
walking boot
Displaced (more common) ▶ urgent ORIF

Sustentaculum tali fxs
Nondisplaced ▶ SLC NWB for 6 wks
> 2 mm displacement ▶ consider ORIF

Diabetic foot ulcers *OKUFA116*

Wagner classification
Grade 0: intact skin (may have bony deformities) ▶ callus
trimming and shoe modification

Grade I: localized superficial ulcer ▶ total contact cast

Grade II: deep ulcer, down to tendon, ligament, bone, or
joint ▶ total contact cast

Grade III: deep abscess and osteomyelitis ▶ debridement,
exostectomy prn

Grade IV: gangrene of toes or forefoot ▶ amputation

Grade V: gangrene of the entire foot ▶ amputation

Navicular fxs *RG2187, BJ2442*

Cortical avulsion fxs: if > 20-25% of articular surface involved
▶ operate

Nondisplaced fxs ▶ SLC for 6-8 wks

Displacement > 2 mm in any plane ▶ ORIF

Lisfranc injuries *RG2203, BJ2441, OKUFA245*

Lisfranc ligament – base of 2nd MT to medial cuneiform
(plantar)

Medial edge of 2nd MT should line up with medial edge of
middle cuneiform

< 1-2 mm stepoff can be normal when aligning medial edge of
4th MT with cuboid

Classification

Homolateral: all 5 MTs displace in same direction

Divergent: displacement of first ray medially, lesser rays
laterally

Displacement (TMT joint widening) > 2 mm or talometatarsal
angle > 15° ▶ ORIF

Cuboid fxs *RG2196*

> 2 mm joint surface disruption or longitudinal compression ▶
ORIF

5th metatarsal fxs *RG2227, OKUFA248*

Zone I: avulsion; if < 2 mm distraction ▶ SLWC or walking
boot; if > 2 mm displaced and > 30% of articular surface ▶
consider ORIF with 4.5 mm screw

Zone II: metaphyseal-diaphyseal junction (Jones fx) ▶ 8-10
wks SLWC (some sources: NWB cast)

Zone III: stress fx of proximal shaft ▶ 6 wks NWB
immobilization vs ORIF; if no healing at 6 weeks ▶ ORIF

1st MTP joint *C3915, OKUFA127*

Normal

ROM: DF = 75°, PF = 35°

MTP (HV) angle ≤ 15° (average: 9°)

Intermetatarsal angle ≤ 9°

DMAA ≤ 10°

Position for great toe arthrodesis *OKUFA132*

10° DF

10-15° valgus

Hallux valgus *OKUFA129*
> Congruent joint
>> ►Chevron, or
>> ► Akin with exostectomy
>
> Incongruent joint
>> IM angle < 13°, HV angle < 30°
>>> ► chevron (age < 50), or
>>> ► distal STP with or without proximal crescentic osteotomy, or
>>> ► Mitchell
>>
>> IM angle ≥ 13°, HV angle < 40°
>>> ► distal STP with proximal crescentic osteotomy, or
>>> ► Mitchell
>>
>> IM angle > 20°, HV angle > 40°
>>> ► distal STP with proximal crescentic osteotomy, or
>>> ► MTP fusion
>
> Hypermobile first ray
>> ► fusion of 1st metatarso-cuneiform joint and distal STP
>
> Degenerative joint disease
>> ► Keller, or
>> ► fusion, or
>> ► prosthesis

MT shaft fxs *RG2222*
> Significant displacement OK medial/lateral
> Beware of dorsal or plantar displacement
> Fxs with > 10° dorsal/plantar deviation or 3-4 mm translation
>> ► correct

Phalangeal fxs *RG2237*
> Gross instability or displaced intra-articular fxs of the interphalangeal joints ► reduction

Turf toe injuries *RG2230*

Sprain of the 1st MTP joint

Grade I: plantar medial tenderness with minimal soft tissue
swelling ▶ conservative tx

Grade II: diffuse tenderness with decreased ROM, moderate
soft tissue swelling ▶ buddy tape for 2 wks

Grade III: severe tenderness, marked soft tissue swelling,
marked decrease ROM ▶ immobilize to limit dorsiflexion

PEDIATRIC TOLERANCES

GENERAL

Synovial fluid analysis *LW468, OKU7-5*
   Findings
      Normal: < 200 leukocytes, < 25% PMNs
      Traumatic: < 5,000 leukocytes with many RBCs, < 25% PMNs
      Toxic synovitis: 5,000-15,000 leukocytes, < 25% PMNs
      Acute rheumatic fever: 10,000-15,000 leukocytes, 50% PMNs
      JRA: 15,000-80,000 leukocytes, 75% PMNs
      Septic arthritis: > 80,000 leukocytes, > 75% PMNs
      Note: there can be considerable variation – one study demonstrated that 55% of bacteriologically proven septic arthritis had < 50,000 WBCs and 34% had < 25,000 WBCs. Also inflammatory diseases (RA) may have counts of > 80,000 WBCs. *(Clin Rheum Dis 1986;12:423)*

DEVELOPMENT & GROWTH

Lower extremity growth *LW55*
   15% proximal femur; 0.6 cm/yr
   37% distal femur; 1.2 cm/yr
   28% proximal tibia; 0.9 cm/yr
   20% distal tibia; 0.7 cm/yr

Upper extremity growth *LW58*
   40% proximal humerus; 1.04 cm/yr
   10% distal humerus; 0.26 cm/yr

10% proximal radius/ulna; 0.25 cm/yr
40% distal radius/ulna; 0.75 cm/yr

Spine growth *LW50*

Spine height equals:
24 cm at infancy
70 cm adult males
65 cm adult females
spinal canal diameter is 95% of adult by 5 yrs

Upper:Lower segment ratio *LW246*

Top of head to superior pubic ramus/superior pubic ramus to
floor
1.6 at birth
0.93 for adults
(helpful for diagnosing disproportionate dwarfism)

General growth parameters *LW35, 223*

Avg growth
25 cm 1st yr of life
10 cm 2nd yr of life
6 cm 3rd and 4th yrs
5 cm/yr thereafter
Height
At 5 y height equals 60% of adult prediction
At 10 y height equals 80% of adult prediction
Diurnal height variation 1.54 cm (range 0.80-2.8 cm)
Weight
Rule of thumb
20 kg at 5 yrs
30 kg at 10 yrs
Puberty
Males 13 yrs
Females 11 yrs

Development & Growth

Leg length discrepancy *LW512,1105, OKUP183, OKU7-472*
>   < 2 cm ► no treatment vs shoe lift if symptomatic
>   2-5 ► shoe lift, contralateral epiphysiodesis vs acute shortenir.g
>   6-20 cm ► leg lengthening (± contralateral shortening if > 8 cm)
>   > 15-20 cm ► consider amp : tation vs VanNess rotationplasty
>   If physeal bridge < 40-50% and accessible with ≥ 2 yrs growth remaining ► excise the physeal bridge (GS134)

Lower extremity alignment *LW72, 110, 1060, OKU7-468*
>   Varus/valgus
>>   10-15° varus at birth
>>   0° varus/valgus 18-24 m
>>   10° valgus (range 2-20°) at 3.5 yrs
>>   6° valgus (range 0-12°) at 6-7 yrs
>   Femoral neck anteversion
>>   Normal = 32° (range 15-50°) at birth
>>   Normal = 16° (range 10-35°) by age 10 yrs
>>   Normal IR of hip = 50° (mid childhood on)
>>   Normal ER of hip = 45° (mid childhood on)
>>   In-toeing children with ≥ 20° ER at hips are normal
>>   Out-toeing children with ≥ 20° IR at hips are normal
>   Tibial torsion
>>   4° external at birth
>>   14° external at 10 yrs
>>   Normal thigh foot angle (TFA) avg = 5° internal (range -30 to +20°) < 8 yrs
>>   Normal TFA avg = 10° internal (range -5 to +30°) ≥ 8 yrs

Development *LW107, 567*
>   Milestones
>>   Head control: 3-6 m
>>   Sitting: 6-9 m

Crawling: 8 m
Pull to stand: 8-12 m
Walking: 12-17 m
Reflexes
Reflexes that disappear
Grasp: 3 m
Moro: 6 m
Asymmetric tonic neck: 6 m
Symmetric tonic neck: 6 m
Neck righting: 10 m
Reflexes that appear
Foot placement: early infancy
Parachute: 12 m
Walking prognosis criteria for CP (*LW577*)
Good
Head balance by 9 m
Independent sitting by 24 m
Crawling by 30 m
Poor
Lack of head balance by 20 m
Inability to sit by 4 yrs

<u>Skeletal Dysplasias</u> *LW247*
Achondroplasia
Kyphosis
If does not correct < 30° on prone hyperextension
radiographs or does not resolve by 3 yrs old (most
resolve) ▶ bracing
If > 40° progressive deformity in child > 5-6 yrs ▶
surgery may be indicated
Chondroectodermal dysplasia
If > 20° ▶ correct genu valgum
see other sections for indications re: scoliosis, AA instability
and coxa vara

HAND

Phalanx fxs *RWB303*

Tolerances – shaft

25° apex volar/dorsal angulation if < 10 yrs old

15° apex volar/dorsal angulation if ≥ 10 yrs old

Abduction/adduction plane remodels less; accept 50% less angulation

20° radial deviation for proximal phalanx IF

20° ulnar deviation for proximal phalanx SF

Expect ~ 10° remodeling in coronal plane in prox phalanx

Expect < 5° of coronal remodeling in middle phalanx

Tolerances – physis

If epiphyseal fragment displaced > 1.5 mm or if 25% of the articular surface is involved ▶ operate

Neck fxs ▶ usually need pinning (unstable)

Metacarpal fxs *RWB328, GS246*

Tolerances

25-35° angulation for SH II fxs, no rotational deformity

10° malrotation for non-physeal MC fxs

20° angulation for basilar thumb MC fxs (some accept 30°)

30-40° angulation for boxer's fxs

Scaphoid fxs *RWB350, OKU7-335*

Tolerance

1 mm displacement

10° angulation

WRIST

Distal radius and ulna *RWB381, GS199, OKU7-334, OKUP111*

Physeal fxs – growth arrest rate = 4-7% for radius, 60% for ulna

Tolerances for 2 yr of growth remaining *(RWB)*
    < 20° deformity
    < 1 mm displacement
Tolerances *(GS)*
    30° angulation if < 10 yrs old
    15° angulation if > 10 yrs old
Metaphyseal fxs
    Tolerances – for the simple minded
        25° in sagittal plane
        10° in frontal plane (radially angulated distal fragment
            should be more readily accepted than an ulnarly
            angulated distal fragment)
    Tolerances – for the mathematically minded
        If ≥ 5 yrs growth remaining:
            Accept 30° angulation in sagittal plane
            Accept 20° angulation in frontal plane
        If < 5 yrs growth remaining:
            4 yrs remaining: accept 25° in sagittal plane
            3 yrs remaining: accept 20° in sagittal plane
            2 yrs remaining: accept 15° in sagittal plane
            (5° less for each yr less of growth remaining)
    Accept 10° malrotation if age ≥ 5 yrs or 15° if age < 5 yrs
    Accept bayonet apposition up to 12 yrs old in the lateral
        plane (≥ 3 yrs growth remaining)
    Accept up to 60% displacement in the frontal plane
Infant greenstick distal forearm fxs
    Tolerances
        ~25° angulation sagittal plane
    Consider CRPP if initial angulation > 30° and disp > 50% or
        if ipsilateral elbow fx is present

FOREARM

Shaft fxs *RWB453. GS204, OKU7-334, OKUP109*

Tolerances

< 8 y/o: 15° angulation, 45° malrotation, complete
displacement, any loss of radial bow

8-14 y/o: 10° angulation, 30° malrotation, complete
displacement, partial loss of radial bow

Indications for operative tx

Unstable fx after closed red

Open fx

Multiple trauma, floating elbow

Refracture with displacement

Compartment syndrome

Segmental/comminuted fx

Accept angulation more readily in distal 1/3 and distal
metaphyseal fxs

Overgrowth is 6-7 mm avg

Monteggia fxs *RWB530*

Bado Classification

Type I: anterior radial head dislocation, diaphyseal ulna fx
▶ flex elbow & supinate

Type II: posterior radial head dislocation, with ulna fx ▶
extend elbow and pronate 45°

Type III: lateral radial head dislocation with ulna fx ▶ flex
elbow and pronate

Type IV: anterior radial head dislocation with radius and
ulna fx ▶ flex elbow

If < 12 yrs old and anatomic radial head reduction with
acceptable (< 10°) angulation of ulna ▶ closed treatment

If closed treatment not possible ▶ percutaneous intramedullary
rods if <12 yrs old or plates if > 12 yrs old

Radial neck fxs *RWB483, GS225, OKU7-303, OKUP102*
  Normal angulation
    AP view 0-15° lateral angulation
    Lat view 10° anterior to 5° posterior angulation (avg 3.5° ant)
  X-ray: radiocapitellar view – beam directed obliquely cephalad from lateral side
  Treatment
    0-30° ▶ simple immobilization
    30-60° ▶ closed manipulation
    If > 45° after closed manipulation ▶ consider percutaneous pin reduction
    If all above methods fail ▶ open reduction ± internal fixation
    Accepting up to 45° angulation generally gives better results than opening
  Tolerances
    < 45° angulation
    ≤ 50% displacement
    ≥ 50-60° of pronation and supination on clinical examination
    ≤ 45-60° angulation if no translation and 60° pronation/supination obtained

ELBOW

Elbow anatomy *RWB564, GS257, OKUP94*
  Normal carrying angle (humeral-ulnar angle)
    0-4 yr old = 15°
    Adult (M = F) = 17.8°
  Ossification
    Capitellum (~2 y): F 1-11 m, M 1-26 m
    Radial head (~4 y): F 3.8 y, M 4.5 y
    Med epicondyle (~6 y): F 5-8 y, M 7-9 y

Trochlea (~8 y): F 7-11 y, M 8-13 y
Olecranon (~9 y): F 6.8 y, M 8.8 y
Lat epicondyle (~11 y): F 8-11 y, M 9-13 y

Baumann's angle – angle of capitellar physis with shaft on AP view

Normal = 73 ± 6°

Anterior humeral line should transect middle 1/3 of capitellum on lat view

Distal humeral condyles normally rotated 5° medially to the shaft

Capitellum normally angulates anteriorly 30-40°

Occult fxs *OKUP93*

Elevation of post fat pad indicates intracapsular fx in > 75% of patients

Radial head subluxation "nursemaid's elbow" *RWB732*

Avg age 2-3 yrs
Females 65%
Left upper extremity 70%
X-rays not necessary with classic history
▶ supinate then flex elbow

Olecranon fxs *RWB520*

< 5 mm displacement (usually stable) ▶ nonoperative treatment
≥ 5 mm displacement and/or instability ▶ ORIF

Coronoid process fxs *RWB525*

Type I   tip ▶ nonoperative
Type II < 50% ▶ nonoperative
Type III > 50% ▶ operative if decreased ROM or instability

Supracondylar humerus fxs *RWB581, OKUP94*

    Peak incidence 5-7 yrs

    6% associated with ipsilateral forearm fx

    Most commonly injured nerve: AIN

    Extension type (98%)

        Type I: nondisplaced, or minimally displaced (ant humeral line still passes through capitellum) ▶ immobilize

        Type II: displaced with posterior cortex intact (fx is stable to external rotation when elbow is flexed to 120°) ▶ CR vs. CRPP if unstable (usually)

        Type III: (posteromedial most common) displaced no cortical contact ▶ CRPP; open if CR not possible

    Tolerances

        Carrying angle must be restored to at least neutral compared to contralateral side

        Accept no varus if normal carrying angle is 0° (avoid cosmetically unacceptable cubitus varus)

        Do not accept > 5° variation of Baumann's angle from opposite side

        Shaft condylar angle (viewed on lat x-ray) should be restored to at least 20° (normal = 30-40°)

        No rotation in horizontal plane

        Anterior humeral line should transect capitellum

        Small amounts of sagittal or coronal translocation are acceptable (remodels easier than angulation)

    Flexion type (2%)

        Type I: minimally displaced < 15-20° increase in shaft condylar angle ▶ immobilize

        Type II: displaced, anterior cortex partially intact ▶ CR vs. CRPP if unstable (usually)

        Type III: totally displaced ▶ often require open reduction

Elbow

Lateral condyle fxs *RWB626, OKUP99*

Milch I: SH IV exits through trochleocapitellar groove

Milch II: more common; SH II exits through trochlea (medial to the lateral condylar ossification center)

Stage I: < 1-2 mm displacement in any plane and articular cartilage surface is intact ▶ splint with very close observation

Stage II: fx line extends through articular cartilage allowing 2-4 mm displacement ▶ tx controversial; usually needs open reduction, although some recommend CRPP if injury is < 48 hrs old and an arthrogram proves that the cartilaginous hinge is intact

Stage III: condylar fragment rotated and totally displaced laterally and proximally ▶ open reduction; beware of cubitus valgus; avoid posterior soft tissue dissection

Capitellum "Mouchet's fx" *RWB647*

Hahn-Steinthal type: includes portion of cancellous bone

Kocher-Lorenz type: pure articular fx may represent a piece of articular cartilage from osteochondritis dessicans (rare in children) ▶ ORIF large fragments; excise small fragments

Medial condylar fxs *RWB651*

Milch type I: fx line traverses apex of trochlea SH II (more common than type II)

Milch type II: fx traverses capitulotrochlear groove SH IV

Kilfoyle's fx displacement patterns

Type I: nondisplaced (incomplete fx line) ▶ posterior splint

Type II: fx extends through cartilage ▶ ORIF if > 2 mm displacement

Type III: condylar fragment both rotated and displaced ▶ ORIF

Beware of cubitus varus and AVN

Fxs of entire distal humeral physis *RWB658, OKUP98*

    Most common in very young children, may occur up to 6 yrs

    Group A: infants 0-12 months, usually SH I

    Group B: children 12 months to 3 yrs (after ossification of
       lateral condylar epiphysis), usually SH I

    Group C: children 3-7 yrs associated with a large metaphyseal
       fragment (most commonly lateral)

    ► CR and immobilization in pronation and flexion; do not
       manipulate if > 5-6 days old

    ► CRPP if significantly disrupted or unstable

Medial epicondyle fxs *RWB672, GS297, OKUP101*

    50% associated with elbow dislocation

    Minimally displaced (< 5 mm) or significantly displaced with
       low demand upper extremity function ► nonoperative

    Operative indications

       Absolute:

          Irreducible incarcerated fragment in elbow joint

       Relative:

          Ulnar nerve dysfunction

          Significant displacement (5-10 mm) with high demand
            upper extremity function

          If the elbow is unstable with > 2 mm displacement of fx

Lateral epicondyle fxs *RWB679*

    Usually nonoperative unless fragment in joint

T-condylar fxs *RWB692*

    Type I: minimally or nondisplaced (<1 mm) ► CRPP

    Type II: displaced no comminution ► CRIF vs. ORIF

    Type III: displaced with comminution ► ORIF

HUMERUS

Humerus diaphyseal fxs *RWB767,GS337*

Tolerances
- 15-30° varus/valgus
- 15-20° ant/post angulation
- 1-2 cm shortening with bayonet apposition
- 15° internal rotation deformity

Usually about 3-12° internal rotation deformity occurs with closed treatment at the expense of ext rotation, however this does not cause functional impairment

Overgrowth occurs in about 80%, usually minimal (< 1 cm)

Clinical appearance is more important than x-ray alignment

Neonatal humeral shaft fxs can remodel 40-50° within 2 yrs

Proximal humerus *RWB745, GS334, OKUP93*

3 growth centers
- Head ossifies at 6 months
- Greater tuberosity ossifies 1-2 years
- Lesser tuberosity ossifies 4-5 years

Tolerances
- < 5 yrs old: 70° angulation; 100% displacement
- 5-12 yrs old: 40-70° angulation
- >12 yrs old: 40° angulation; 50% displacement
- Reduction may not be indicated unless patient is within 2 yrs of maturity and angulation > 25° ▶ tx with sling and swath

Neer-Horwitz classification and recommendations
- Grade I: < 5 mm displacement ▶ sling & swath without reduction
- Grade II: < 1/3 shaft width ▶ sling and swath without reduction
- Grade III: 2/3 shaft width ▶ reduce if angulation is severe

Grade IV: > 2/3 shaft width ▶ reduce and apply salute
position spica (may be a little outdated for modern times)
Thoracobrachial dressing (coaptation splint, sling and swathe,
or a commercial shoulder immobilizer), or occasionally a
hanging arm cast in older children are all considered
acceptable forms of tx.
> 12 years old with markedly displaced fx ▶ CRPP
Most physeal injuries through 5 yrs of age are SH I and do not
require anatomic reduction
Lesser tuberosity fxs in athletes ▶ repair
Greater tuberosity fxs ▶ reduce and immobilize vs. ORIF per
adult indications
Most epiphyseal fxs are stable by 2-3 wks
Most metaphyseal fxs stable by 3-4 wks
Birth injuries heal by 2-3 wks

SHOULDER GIRDLE

Clavicle fxs *RWB762*
True AC dislocation does not occur in children < 13 yrs
(physeal fx)
Nonoperative treatment for most distal clavicle fxs and AC
separations in children < 16 yrs old
Obstetric midshaft fxs ▶ nonoperative treatment

Glenoid fxs *RWB756*
Operate if shoulder unstable and large part of glenoid involved,
ie:
> 25% ant surface or 33% post surface
> 5 mm articular stepoff

SPINE

C-spine *RWB816, GS344, OKU7-589, OKUSpine116, OKUP134, LW801*

Radiography

Atlanto-dens interval (ADI) up to 5 mm may be normal

Space available for the cord (SAC) should be $\geq$ 13 mm

C1-C2 facet joint angles:

Shallow at birth (~55°)

Increase to 70° by age 8

Lower c-spine facet joint angles = 30° in neonates and 65° in adults

Odontoid normally directly below basion (5 mm avg distance)

in infants and small children up to 1 cm can be normal

If > 1-2 cm ▶ evaluate

Os odontoidium normally moves < 3 mm

Symptomatic os odontoidium may move up to 1 cm

Pseudosubluxation

Anterior displacement of C2 on C3 of $\leq$ 4 mm or C3 on C4 $\leq$ 3 mm may be normal

Differentiated from pathologic subluxation by the posterior cervical line (Swischuk) drawn from the anterior cortex of the C1 posterior arch to the anterior cortex of the C3 posterior arch. The anterior cortex of the C2 posterior arch should lie within 1 mm of this line. If $\geq$ 1.5 mm, then suspect pathologic C2-3 subluxation.

Suspect soft tissue injury if > 10 mm widening between spinous processes of C1-C2

Retropharyngeal soft tissues > 7 mm at C2 base and > 14 mm at the base of C6 is abnormal

Torg ratio (canal to vertebral body) $\geq$ 0.8

Hangman's fx – spondylolistheses of C2

► gentle reduction and halo or Minerva cast

Delayed union with instability or nonunion ► surgery

AA instability in Down's syndrome

> 5 mm ► restrict from sports, operate if symptomatic (controversial)

SAC < 10 mm ► fuse

Rotary displacement – rarely associated with neurologic findings

Classification

Type I: simple rotary displacement no anterior shift of C1

Type II: rotary displacement with anterior shift of ≤ 5 mm (anterior displacement of > 4 mm in young children or > 3 mm in older children/adults is considered pathologic)

Type III: rotary displacement with anterior shift > 5 mm

Type IV: rotary displacement with posterior shift

Treatment

If < 1 wk ► soft collar/analgesics and close follow up

If < 1 wk < 1 month ► hospitalize/halter traction/muscle relaxants then Minerva collar x 6 wks following reduction if there was anterior if anterior displacement; if < 4 y/o halo required due to patient noncompliance

If > 1 month ► hospitalize/halo and traction if reduction fails or > 3 months ► fusion

TLS-spine

Normal thoracic kyphosis = 10-40° T5-12

Normal lumbar lordosis = 30-60° T12-S1

Scheurmann's kyphosis *OKUP14, LW323, 754*

Criteria: > 3 consecutive vertebra with ≥ 5° anterior wedging each

Spine

Treatment
If > 50-70° ▶ brace
If ≥ 75° ▶ consider operation
Congenital scoliosis/kyphosis *LW55, OKUP317, LW727*
Block or wedge vertebrae (curve progression usually 0-2° per yr) ▶ PSIF if progressive
Hemivertebra (curve progression usually 1-3.5° per yr for each hemivertebra) ▶ observation vs hemiepiphysiodesis vs excision
Unilateral unsegmented bar (curve progression usually 6-9° per year, slightly less for upper thoracic) ▶ spinal fusion required
Unilateral unsegmented bar with contralateral HV (curve progression usually > 10° per yr, slightly less for upper thoracic and thoracic) ▶ spinal fusion required
Lumbosacral hemivertebra with trunk decompensation ▶ hemivertebra excision (controversial)
Convex hemiarthrodesis/epiphysiodesis indicated for curves < 50° in children < 5 yrs
Correction of up to 10-15° can be obtained with hemiepiphysiodesis during first 5 yrs
Kyphosis < 5 yrs with < 50-55° ▶ posterior fusion alone
Kyphosis > 55° ▶ anterior and posterior fusion
Duchenne's muscular dystrophy *OKUP270, LW641*
95% develop progressive scoliosis
Curves 20-30° ▶ PSIF to L5 (FVC ≥ 30-40% predicted)
Curves > 40° or pelvic obliquity > 10° ▶ PSIF to the pelvis (FVC ≥ 30-40% predicted)
Spinal muscular atrophy (SMA) *OKUP273*
PSIF for curves > 40° (FVC ≥ 30-40% predicted)
Neuromuscular scoliosis *OKUP281, LW570*
15% of brace treated curves stop progressing
Curves < 25-30° ▶ observation
Curves 25-40° ▶ bracing

Curves > 40-45° ▶ operate (if cognitive function and
  comorbidities allow)
Rigid curves not correcting to < 50-60° on bending films
  may require anterior fusion
LS obliquity > 15° ▶ fuse to pelvis
Infantile idiopathic scoliosis *LW694*
Rib vertebral angle difference (RVAD) > 20° predicts likely
  (84%) progression
Adolescent idiopathic scoliosis *OKUP287, LW677*
Cobb angle of > 10° required to establish the diagnosis
Scoliometer reading (trunk rotation) ≥ 7° ▶ referral for
  radiographic workup
Cobb angle interobserver variability = 7.2°
Cobb angle intraobserver variability = 4.9°
Progression of 10° required to be 95% confident of true
  progression
Diurnal variation = 5° average curve increase in pm
Risser staging (ossification of iliac apophysis)
  Grade I: lateral 25% ossified
  Grade II: lateral 50% ossified
  Grade III: lateral 75% ossified
  Grade IV: 100% ossified (corresponds with completion
    of spinal growth)
  Grade V: fusion of iliac apophysis
Risk of progression
  Risser 0-1
    = 22% of curves 5-19° will progress
    = 68% for curves 20-29° will progress
    = 90% for curves 30-59° will progress
  At maturity
    68% of curves > 50° will progress
    thoracic curves 50-75° progress about 1° per yr
    curves < 30° tend not to progress

Pulmonary function decreases when thoracic curves approach 100°

Classification (Lenke)

Curve type (1-6) + Lumbar spine modifier (A, B, C) + Thoracic sagittal modifier (-, N, +); example: 1B+; see below

Major = largest curve (Cobb), always structural

Curve type

1: main thoracic (MT major)

2: double thoracic (MT major)

3: double major (MT major)

4: triple major (MT major)

5: thoracolumbar/lumbar (TL/L major)

6: thoracolumbar/lumbar – main thoracic (TL/L major)

Structural Criteria (Minor curves)

Proximal thoracic: side bending Cobb ≥ 25° or T2-T5 kyphosis ≥ +20°

Main thoracic: side bending Cobb ≥ 25° or T10-L2 kyphosis ≥ +20°

Thoracolumbar/lumbar: side bending Cobb ≥ 25° or T10-L2 kyphosis ≥ +20°

Lumbar spine modifier

A: CSVL between pedicles

B: CSVL touches apical pedicle(s)

C: CSVL completely medial

Thoracic sagittal profile T5-T12

Hypo (-): < 10°

Normal (N): 10-40°

Hyper (+): > 40°

Location of apex

Thoracic: apex T12 to T11/12 disc

Thoracolumbar: T12 to L1

Lumbar: L1/2 disc to L4

Treatment
Skeletally immature (Risser 0-2)
Curves 20-40° ▶ bracing (30-50% risk of
progression in brace), some surgeons prefer to
demonstrate progression > 5° prior to initiation of
bracing for curves < 30°
Curves 40-50° or curve progression despite bracing
▶ PSIF
Anterior approach recommended for:
Age < 10 yrs (Risser ≤ 1, triradiate open)
Skeletally mature
Thoracic curves > 50° ▶ PSIF
Thoracolumbar/lumbar curves > 40° (especially with
marked trunk rotation)
Classification
Spondylolisthesis *OKUP329, LW782*
Meyerding grading system (L5 on S1)
Grade I: 1-25% slip ▶ nonoperative mgmt; if fails ▶
operate
Grade II: 26-50% slip ▶ nonoperative mgmt; if fails ▶
operate
Grade III: 51-75% slip ▶ operate
Grade IV: 76-100% slip ▶ operate
Grade V: > 100% slip ▶ operate
Slip angles > 45° have high risk of progression
Chance fx – flexion distraction injury *RWB860*
Usually L1-L3 in children (T-L junction in adults)
If truly bony in all columns ▶ hyperextension TLSO or
Risser cast if kyphosis < 20°
If ligamentous ▶ compression rod

PELVIS AND ACETABULUM

Pelvis *GS383*
Open book < 3 cm symphyseal separation ▶ bedrest
Ischial tuberosity apophyseal avulsion ▶ ORIF if displaced > 2 cm

Acetabulum *GS387*
< 1 mm displacement ▶ bedrest or NWB
1-2 mm displacement ▶ traction
≥ 2 mm displacement ▶ ORIF
Nonoperative treatment duration
    4-6 wks if < 7 yrs
    6-8 wks if 7-14 yrs
    8-12 wks if > 14 yrs

HIP

Septic hip *LW475*
Parameters
    Serum WBC > 11,000
    Temperature > 101.0
    Unable to weight bear
    ESR > 40
Probability
    4/4 parameters present 99%
    3/4 parameters present 95%
    2/4 parameters present 50%

Fxs of the hip *RWB914, GS389, OKUP81*
Delbet classification
    Type I: transepiphyseal separation ▶ open vs. closed reduction and smooth Steinmann pin fixation
    Type II: transcervical fxs (most common), AVN rate up to 50% ▶ open reduction and pin or screw fixation

Type III: cervicotrochanteric fxs, AVN rate 20-30% ▶ open reduction and pin or screw fixation

Type IV: intertrochanteric fxs ▶ CRPP or ORIF, reduce to within 5° of normal neck shaft angle

Vascular supply to the femoral head

ligamentum teres contributes 20% in adults but very little before 8 yrs old

metaphyseal supply becomes nonexistent by age 4 and comes from medial and lateral circumflex arteries

lateral epiphyseal vessels – bypass physis & become more important later in life; originate from MFC artery posterior superior branch (dominates after age 3-4) and posterior inferior branch

Increased femoral anteversion *OKUP22*

Internal rotation of hip > 70° = increased femoral anteversion

If ≥ 80° IR, < 10° ER, and/or CT shows ≥ 50° femoral anteversion ▶ consider derotation osteotomy

Cerebral palsy hip *LW574, OKUP242*

Migration index (MI) of Reimers – the percentage of the femoral head that lies outside (beyond Perkin's line) the acetabulum

Hip at risk – hips with < 30° abduction or > 20° flexion contracture or with break in Shenton's line

If MI < 30% ▶ adductor release (do not do anterior obturator neurectomy in ambulators or as an initial procedure. If < 6 yrs consider Botox treatment.

Subluxation

If MI = 30-50% ▶ adductor tenotomy and VDRO (should obtain ≥ 50-60° abduction intraoperatively)

If MI > 50% ▶ open reduction/capsulorrhaphy, adductor tenotomy, and VDRO

If hip flexion contracture > 15° ► add iliopsoas tenotomy at pelvic brim

If acetabular index is > 25° ► add pelvic osteotomy unless very young

X-ray hips Q6 months in nonambulators during growth spurt and/or if loosing abduction

Developmental dysplasia of the hip (DDH) *LW905, OKUP161*

Normal
  Newborn
    Male: 26°
    Female: 28°
  6 m
    Male: 21°
    Female: 23°
  12 m
    Male: 21°
    Female: 22°

Age 0-6 months ► Pavlik if not reducing discontinue before 3 wks

Age 6 months – 2 yrs ► CR and cast vs open reduction

Age > 18 – 24 months ► add pelvic and femoral osteotomies

Developmental coxa vara *LW1040*

Normal Hilgenreiner-physeal (HP) angle = 25°

If HP angle > 45-60° ► valgus osteotomy and attempt neck shaft angle of > 160° (93% of osteotomies with residual HP angle > 40° will result in recurrence)

Legg Calve Perthes disease *LW957, OKUP153*

Most common ages 4-8 yrs

Bilateral 10%

Classification
  Salter Thompson

    A: crescent sign involves < ½ of the epiphysis (Catterall
      I & II)
    B: crescent sign involves > ½ of the epiphysis with
      lateral pillar fragmentation (Catterall III & IV)
Herring – lateral pillar classification
    A: no lateral pillar involvement
    B: > 50% height of lateral pillar maintained
    B/C border: 50% height of lateral pillar maintained
    C: < 50% height of lateral pillar maintained
Lateral extrusion of > 20% of the epiphysis & age > 8 yrs at the
    time of onset correlates with poor prognosis
Treatment – controversial
    Recent multicenter prospective trial shows the following
      results (*Herring, JBJS 86-A:Oct 2004;2121*)
      Chronologic age ≤ 8.0 yrs (skeletal age ≤ 6.0 yrs) at
        onset ▶ no treatment (observation, operative and
        nonoperative txs all had equivalent results)
      Chronologic age > 8.0 yrs at onset with lateral pillar
        group B or B/C border ▶ operative tx (improved
        outcomes compared to nonoperative)
      Chronologic age > 8.0 yrs at onset with lateral pillar
        group C and/or physeal extrusion > 20% does poorly
        regardless of tx

Slipped capital femoral epiphysis *LW999, OKUP143*
    Most common ages 10-14 yrs
    Bilateral approximately 30%
    Radiography: Klein's line does not transect lateral portion of
      the epiphysis
    Treatment
      ▶ single pin fixation in center of head, tip not closer than 5
        mm to articular surface
    Up to 50% osteonecrosis in unstable slips

FEMUR

Femoral shaft fxs *RWB948, GS407, OKUP85*

Tolerances

0-2 years: 30° varus/valgus; 30° AP angulation; 15 mm shortening

2-5 years: 15° varus/valgus; 20° AP angulation; 20 mm shortening

6-10 years: 10° varus/valgus; 15° AP angulation; 15 mm shortening

≥ 11 years: 5° varus/valgus; 10° AP angulation; 10 mm shortening

All ages: ≤ 10° malrotation

*≤ 2.5 cm shortening accepted on follow-up exam for ages 2-10 yrs

Treatment

0-6 months

Stable fx ► splint or Pavlik harness

Unstable fx ► (angulation > 30° or > 1-2 cm shortening
► immediate spica or modified Bryant's then spica

6 months – 5 yrs

Stable or unstable < 3 cm initial shortening (neg telescope test) ► 90/90 spica

If > 3 cm initial shortening (some say 1.5 cm) or if obese
► 7-10 days traction then spica

6-11 yrs

stable ► flexible nails vs. immediate spica

unstable ► flexible nails vs. 90/90 traction then spica

≥ 12 yrs

► consider locked IMR with trochanteric entry

Spica casting

Increase flexion and abduction for proximal fxs

Proximal 1/3 fxs ► flex hip 45-90° abduct 30° and ER 15°

Middle 1/3 fxs ► flex hip 30° abduct 15° and ER 15°
Distal 1/3 fxs ► full hip extension and ER 15°
Average overgrowth
  < 10 yrs old = 9 mm (range 4-25 mm)
  78% occurs in the first 18 months

Supracondylar femur fxs/distal femoral physeal fxs *RWB992,*
  OKUP89
  Tolerances
    5-10° varus/valgus angulation*
    10-20° AP angulation* (Blount states that ≤ 20° posterior
      angulation can be accepted without developing a
      recurvatum deformity in younger patients)
    *Higher end of range accepted only in younger ages
    Anatomic reduction necessary for SH III or IV injuries
  Treatment
    If unstable/displaced ► smooth transphyseal crossed pins or
      metaphyseal screws if Thurston-Holland fragment > 2.5
      cm
    ~25-40% of significant distal femoral physeal injuries will
      develop deformities/shortening
    Growth plate deformity ► excise bony bridge if < 25-50% of
      growth plate involved and > 2 yrs of growth remain

Proximal Femoral Focal Deficiency *LW1236*
    Aitken Classification
    Class A: femoral head-present, femoral segment-short,
      subtroch varus, acetabulum-normal
    Class B: femoral head-present, femoral segment-short, no
      prox osseous connection, acetabulum-normal
    Class C: femoral head-absent, femoral segment-short,
      proximally tapered, acetabulum-dysplastic

Class D: femoral head-absent, femoral segment- short
   irregularly ossified tuft, acetabulum-absent, flat lateral
   pelvic wall

KNEE

Patella fxs *RWB1033*
   Displacement > 3mm (stepoff or diastasis) ▶ ORIF
   Marginal fxs ▶ excise
   Osteochondral fragment > 1 cm ▶ ORIF

Bipartite patella *OKUP192*
   Type I inferior pole 5%
   Type II entire lateral margin 20%
   Type III superior lateral corner 75%
   Treatment
      Acute injuries ▶ immobilize
      Chronic pain ▶ excise for chronic pain

Patellar dislocation *RWB1060*
   Normal Q angle
      Boys = 10°
      Girls = 15°
   Recurrence rates
      < 11 yrs: 15-20%
      11-14 yrs: 60%
      19-28 yrs: 30%

Meniscal tears *RWB1065*
   Peripheral tears < 1 cm ▶ cast immobilization for 6-8 wks
   MRI shows 55% false positive meniscus tear rate in children <
      15 yrs

Tibial tubercle avulsion fxs *RWB1023, OKUP119*
- Ogden Classification
  - Type I: fx through tib tubercle distal to horizontal portion of the physis
  - Type II: fx through tib tubercle exiting anteriorly at/above the horizontal physis
  - Type III: fx propagates intraarticular
- Operative treatment indicated for all but the smallest fragments
- Patient must have full active extension for nonoperative treatment
- ~10% of proximal tibial physeal injuries will develop growth disturbance

Knee osteochondral fxs *OKU7-474, RWB1037*
- If > 2 cm or if ≥ 1 cm with a larger osseus component ▶ operate
- May have a lower threshold for operating if on a weight bearing surface

Flexion contractures *OKUP279, LW587*
- Arthrogryposis
  - Flexion contracture < 20° ▶ stretching
  - Flexion contracture 20-40° ▶ hamstring lengthening
  - Moderate contractures ≤ 50° ▶ may require z-plasty/serial casting
  - Severe contractures 60-80° ▶ gradual correction with ex-fix +/- femoral shortening
- Cerebral Palsy
  - Popliteal angle <135° (cannot extend beyond 45° with hip flexed 90°) ▶ hamstring lengthening (should increase popliteal angle to ≥ 160° intraoperatively)

Discoid meniscus *OKUP193*

    Watanabe classification

        Type I: stable thickened disc complete ▶ arthroscopic sculpting

        Type II: stable thickened disc incomplete ▶ arthroscopic sculpting

        Type III: normal shape thickened posterior horn (Wrisberg variant) ▶ capsular suture

Popliteal cyst (Baker's cyst) *OKUP198*

    70% resolve in pediatric patients within 12-24 months

    30-40% recurrence rate with surgery

Tibial spine (eminence) fxs *RWB1040, GS452, OKU7-473, OKUP117*

    Meyers-McKeever Classification

        Type I: minimal displacement ▶ possible aspiration then cast x 6 wks in neutral to 10° flexion

        Type II: anterior portion displaced with posterior hinge ▶ treatment as in type I vs. fixation if unreducible

        Type III: complete separation ▶ operative fixation

Ligament sprains *RWB1045, LW1290*

    1st degree minimum number of fibers torn, no instability; ≤ 5 mm joint surface separation

    2nd degree more torn fibers causing loss of function but no significant instability; 5-10 mm joint surface separation

    3rd degree complete disruption of the ligament resulting in instability in the knee; > 10 mm joint separation

Congenital knee dislocation *LW1095, OKUP192*

    Type I (hyperextended knee) ▶ resolves

    Type II (tibial subluxation) ▶ serial casting

Type III (tibial dislocation) or failure of nonop management of
types I or II to obtain ≥ 60° flexion ▶ surgical
reduction/quadricepsplasty

<u>ACL rupture *OKU7-473*</u>
If > 2 cm growth remaining in the knee ▶ nonsurgical
treatment vs. extraphyseal reconstruction
If < 2 cm growth remaining ▶ hamstring graft through
anatomic bony tunnels
If near maturity ▶ bone-patellar tendon-bone autograft vs.
hamstrings graft

TIBIA AND FIBULA

<u>Tibia fxs *RWB1094, GS472, OKU7-475, OKUP121*</u>
Proximal metaphyseal
Most common age 3-8 yrs
Valgus deformity common sequela (peaks at 12-18 months
post fx) but > 90% correct on their own
Chronic residual valgus > 20° ▶ consider osteotomy (or
hemiepiphysiodesis if > 15°)
Diaphyseal
30% of shaft fxs in children are associated with ipsilateral
fibular fx (without fibular fx tend to go into varus)
Tolerances (*RWB*)
If < 8 years
5° valgus
10° varus
10° ant angulation
5° post angulation
10 mm shortening
5° rotation
If ≥ 8 years
5° valgus
5° varus

            5° ant angulation
            0° post angulation
            5 mm shortening
            5° rotation
    Tolerances (*OKU/OKUP*)
        Don't accept any valgus
        If < 8 yrs may accept up to 10° varus and 50% apposition
        Maximum 1 cm shortening
    Tolerances (*GS*)
        Varus deformity up to 15° (will remodel)
        Valgus deformities tend to persist
        Females 3-10 yrs – shortening 5-10 mm
        Males 3-12 yrs – shortening 5-10 mm
    Average overgrowth is about 4 mm

Toddler's fx *RWB1108*
    Spiral fx of tibia (no fibula fx) – avg age = 27 months
    ▶ long leg cast with knee flexion for 2-3 wks, then SLWC for
      2 wks

Tibial stress fx *RWB1113*
    Usually proximal 1/3
    Peak incidence 10-15 yrs
    Treatment: activity modification or LLC for 4-6 wks

Distal tibia *RWB1142, GS524, OKU7-476, OKUP125*
    Distal physis ossification center appears at 6-24 months, with
      malleolar extension ~7 years
    Physis closes ~15 yrs in females; 17 yrs in males
    Closure takes ~18 months; begins centrally then proceeds
      medially then laterally
    Tolerances – distal physis
      SH I & II

All ages: ≥ 3 mm residual gap anteriorly at physis
indicates entrapped periosteum & should be opened
to prevent physeal arrest
> 2 yrs growth remaining
15° plantar tilt for posteriorly displaced fxs
10° valgus for laterally displaced fxs
0° varus for medially displaced fxs
< 2 yrs growth remaining
< 5° angulation in all planes
Angular deformity secondary to malunion if < 20° ▶
wait 2 yrs for remodeling then do supramalleolar
osteotomy if residual varus/valgus > 20°
SH III & IV
< 1 mm displacement or < 2 mm gap ▶ nonoperative
> 2 mm displacement ▶ ORIF
1-2 mm displacement ▶ CR in operating room, possible
CRPP
If seen > 7 days post injury accept up to 2 mm without
attempting any reduction

___

Blount's disease *LW1066, OKUP23*
See LE alignment in beginning of pediatric section
Metaphyseal diaphyseal (MD) angle
< 11° is normal
> 16° predicts development of Blount's
11-16° monitor closely
Treatment
2-3 yrs ▶ single medial upright brace with locked knee &
valgus strap
If no resolution or Langenskold stage III ▶ valgus
osteotomy indicated by age 4 yrs (overcorrect to 5-10°
valgus)

ANKLE

Fibular physeal fxs *RWB1146*
  Nondisplaced ▶ SLWC 3-4 wks
  Displaced ▶ reduce, (may accept ≤ 50% displacement)

Tib-fib overlap
  Appears on mortise view at:
    Females: age 10 y
    Males: age 16 y

Juvenile tilleaux fxs *RWB1147*
  External rotation fx of anterior-lateral distal tibia, fragment is
    avulsed by ant-inf tibiofibular ligament
  If displaced < 2 mm ▶ LLC with knee flexed 30° and foot
    internally rotated, confirm reduction with post reduction CT
    scan
  If displaced > 2 mm ▶ CR possible percutaneous pinning

Triplane fxs *RWB1152, OKU7-543, GS531*
  Posterior metaphyseal spike (SH II)
  Anterolateral epiphyseal fragment (SH III)
  Tolerances
    < 2 mm displaced ▶ immobilize and confirm with CT scan;
      LLC with knee flexed to 30-40°, with foot int rot for lat
      fxs, eversion for medial fxs.
    > 2 mm displaced ▶ closed vs. open reduction possible
      percutaneous or internal fixation
    > 3 mm displaced usually requires ORIF (closed reduction
      difficult)
    Do not accept > 3 mm interfragmentary gap (in contrast to
      step-off)

FOOT

Thigh foot angle (TFA) *OKUP22*
    TFA slightly medial at birth corrects over time to 10° lateral
        (range 0-20°)
    Normal foot progression angle 1-4 yrs = 40° inward – 40°
        outward
    Surgical indications (late childhood)
        Medial TFA ≥ 10°
        Lateral TFA ≥ 35°

Talar neck fxs *RWB1174*
    Tolerances
        1-5 mm displacement
        < 5° angulation
    AVN rates
        Type I: 0%
        Type II: 40%
        Type III: 90%

Calcaneal fxs *RWB1193*
    Extra-articular nondisplaced ▶ WBAT usually OK especially
        if young
    Adolescents with displaced fxs ▶ treat as an adult

TMT dislocation *RWB1197*
    Minimal displacement (≤ 2-3 mm) ▶ elevation until swelling
        subsides then cast for 2-4 wks
    > 2-3 mm displacement ▶ CR vs. open reduction possible
        percutaneous pins

MT fxs *RWB1199*

    Neck most common location

    Considerable degree of lateral displacement can be accepted
and moderate amounts of dorsal angulation of MT necks
will remodel in a child

    Avulsion at the base of the 5th MT – apophysis usually not
present before age 8 ▶ SLWC x 3-6 wks

    Jones fx – metaphyseal-diaphyseal junction (not an avulsion
mechanism) acute ▶ trial of NWB cast

        Repetitive symptoms or intramedullary sclerosis – prognosis
poor without operative intervention ▶ usually
intramedullary screw

        Stress fxs ▶ cast x 2 wks

    Acute tuberosity avulsion fxs with > 3 mm displacement in
young active pt with an unusually long tuberosity ▶
operative fixation

Phalanx fxs *GS564*

    Great toe proximal phalanx

    If > 30 % of articular surface involved or > 3 mm displacement
▶ ORIF

Tarsal coalition *LW1185*

    Calcaneonavicular & talocalcaneal are most common

    Only 25% of pts with tarsal coalition become symptomatic

    Onset of pain 8-12 yrs for calcaneonavicular coalition

    Onset of pain 12-16 yrs for talocalcaneal coalition

    Poor results reported if resection of a talocalcaneal coalition
involving > 50% of posterior facet

Clubfoot *OKUP204*
> Radiography
> > Talocalcaneal angle < 20° on AP view indicates hindfoot
> > > varus
> > Talocalcaneal angle < 35° on lat view indicates equinus
> > Talo-1st MT angle > 0° on AP view indicates adductus
> > Tibiocalcaneal angle > 90° on forced dorsiflexion confirms
> > > equinus contracture

APPENDIX

ORDERING INFORMATION

For further questions, or to place an order, please contact:

Peggy Stark
G. Mosser Taylor Memorial Library
Department of Orthopaedic Surgery
Loma Linda University
11406 Loma Linda Drive, Suite 218
Loma Linda, CA 92354
e-mail: pstark@llu.edu
phone: (909) 558-6444, ext. 62708

ABBREVIATIONS

AA	atlanto-axial		LC	lateral compression
abd	abduction		L-C	lunate-capitate
ABI	ankle brachial index		LF	long finger
abx	antibiotics		LLC	long leg cast
AC	acromioclavicular		LP	length of patella
ACL	anterior cruciate ligament		LT	length of tendon
add	adduction		MC	metacarpal
ADI	atlanto-dens interval		MCL	medial collateral ligament
ALL	anterior longitudinal ligament		MFC	medial femoral condyle
ant	anterior		MP	metacarpophalangeal
AO	atlanto-occipital		MT	metatarsal
AP	anteroposterior		MTP	metatarsophalangeal
APC	anteroposterior compression		nl	normal
ATFL	anterior talofibular ligament		NWB	non-weightbearing
avg	average		ON	osteonecrosis
AVN	avascular necrosis		ORIF	open reduction internal fixation
CC	coracoclavicular		PCL	posterior cruciate ligament
CFL	calcaneofibular ligament		PF	plantarflexion
CM	combination		PIN	posterior interosseous nerve
CMC	carpometacarpal		PIP	proximal interphalangeal
CR	closed reduction		PLC	posterolateral corner
CRPP	closed reduction perc pinning		PLL	posterior longitudinal ligament
CTLSO	cervico-thoraco-lumbo-sacral orthosis		post	posterior
DBP	diastolic blood pressure		prox	proximal
DDD	degenerative disk disease		PSIF	post spinal instrumentation & fusion
DF	dorsiflexion		RCL	radial collateral ligament
DIP	distal interphalangeal		RCT	rotator cuff tear
DISI	dorsal intercalated segment instability		RF	ring finger
disp	displacement		ROM	range of motion
dist	distal		R-S	radioscaphoid
DJD	degenerative joint disease		SAC	space available for cord
DMMA	distal metatarsal articular angle		SC	sternoclavicular
DRUJ	distal radial-ulnar joint		SF	small finger
dz	disease		SH	Salter-Harris
EIF	extended iliofemoral		S-L	scapholunate
ER	external rotation		SLAP	superior labrum anterior-posterior
ext	extension		SLD	scapholunate dissociation
f/u	follow-up		SLR	straight leg raise
flex	flexion		SLWC	short leg walking cast
fx	fracture		STP	soft tissue procedure
GSW	gun shot wound		TFCC	triangular fibrocartilage complex
HTLSO	hip-thoraco-lumbo-sacral orthosis		THA	total hip arthroplasty
HV	hallux valgus		TLSO	thoraco-lumbo-sacral orthosis
IF	index finger		TMT	tarsometatarsal
IM	intermetatarsal		UCL	ulnar collateral ligament
IMR	intramedullary rodding		VISI	volar intercalated segment instability
IR	internal rotation		VS	vertical shear
lat	lateral		WBAT	weight bearing as tolerate